Head and Neck Anatomy:
An Introduction and Laboratory Guide

David W. Brzezinski, M.D.

ISBN: 1499652127
ISBN-13: 978-1499652123

ACKNOWLEDGMENTS

The author would like to formally thank the faculty members at the University of Michigan Division of Anatomical Sciences for their feedback during the development of this text. In particular, Drs. Jerry Cortright, John Stribley, Kelli Sullivan, Kathleen Alsup and Glenn Fox provided great assistance.

The author would also like to thank Drs. Tom Gest and Ameed Raoof for sparking his interest in human gross anatomy and for laying the foundations of its understanding.

Additionally, the author would like to thank Drs. Jerry Cortright and Walter Castelli for their mentorship in head and neck anatomy over the course of many years.

Finally, the author would like to recognize the electronic MedCharts (by Gest and Schlesinger, et. al.) and the Laboratory and Study Guide for Head and Neck Anatomy: Dissection of the Head and Neck (by Brzezinski and Cortright, et. al.). These works were critical to the author's understanding and arrangement of the materials contained within this text.

AUTHOR'S NOTE REGARDING REVISIONS

In editing the first printings of this text it was noticed that certain citing omissions occurred. These have been corrected in this updated version.

CONTENTS

Introduction

The study of human gross anatomy is an amazing privilege, and a unique one as well. The student of gross anatomy should appreciate this from the beginning of his or her studies. Very few people ever have the opportunity to study the human body in great detail.

Unlike many, if not most, other academic endeavors, the study of human gross anatomy is a very visual undertaking. Instead of memorizing a list of facts, the study of human gross anatomy requires the student to memorize the arrangement of three-dimensional structures which collectively create one large three-dimensional structure (the human body). One may think of this as the construction of a puzzle within one's mind. The successful study of gross anatomy, therefore, requires the student to be able to reconstruct the entire human body in a three-dimensional fashion.

The arrangement of the human body consists of the collection of smaller and smaller subunits which function together as a whole (the organism). Therefore, atoms combine to create molecules. Molecules combine to create cellular machinery and organelles. Cellular machinery and organelles combine to create cells. Cells combine to create tissues. Tissues combine to create organs. Organs combine to create organ systems. Finally, organ systems combine and work together to create the organism. Human gross anatomy studies the organ, organ systems, and the human body as a whole. Smaller subunits are studied in other disciplines such as histology and cellular and molecular biology.

Head and neck anatomy, the domain of certain physicians, surgeons, and dental professionals, is the specific study of the head and neck region of the human body. There are many ways to approach the study of human anatomy, and head and neck anatomy in particular. Over many years of teaching medical and dental students and medical and dental residents, the author of this text has come to appreciate the fact that students all learn in unique ways. This being said, however, certain methods seem best suited to the majority of students. Dissection is a large part of these methods. As such, this text is intended as an adjunct to study of the human body in the dissection laboratory. Ideally, the student will study the head and neck in a regional manner with an anatomy atlas (with images), this text (with descriptions of important regional structures), and with the cadaver in the laboratory setting.

This text is not intended to be an exhaustive account of the entire head and neck. Instead, the author has created it as a brief introduction to the region to be used as the student studies the human cadaver and relevant regional imagery in an atlas or other resource. The author of this text also realizes that he is not infallible and is prone to error. The human body, however, never makes an error. There may be (and in fact will be) variation from body to body. But, "it is what it is", to borrow the idiom. The human cadaver, therefore, is the student's best source of information on the arrangement of the human body.

In undertaking the teaching of human gross anatomy, the author (and likely nearly every other instructor) writes, lectures, and instructs in a manner which assumes the student is familiar with basic anatomic terminology. Clearly the beginning student has no such familiarity with said terminology. Therefore, some important anatomic terms are briefly defined here following this introduction. The student should take the time to memorize these terms before doing any other study of the human body. It will make the subsequent reading of this text (and any other gross anatomy resources) possible, meaningful and even enjoyable.

\-   David W. Brzezinski, M.D.
May, 2014

Key Terminology

Descriptive Anatomy: the physical description of structures within the body (including size, shape, color, etc.), contextual relationships (deep, superficial, medial, lateral, anterior, posterior, etc.), and names of said structures. (1, p. 11)

Functional Anatomy: the morphologic basis for the role played by structures in the normal functioning of the body. This is the domain of present day physiology, but originally physiology was a subdiscipline of gross anatomy. (2, p. 11)

Regional Anatomy: the study of regions or specific areas of the body. Examples include the head, neck, thorax, abdomen, pelvis, perineum and limbs. This text is organized in a regional approach. (3, p. 11)

Systemic Anatomy: the study of structures grouped together morphologically and/or functionally within specific organ systems of the body. Examples include the cardiovascular system, pulmonary system, nervous system, endocrine system, musculoskeletal system, gastrointestinal system, genitourinary system, integumentary system, lymphatic system, etc. (4, p. 11)

Planes of the body:

> Sagittal plane: this plane is named after the sagittal suture of the skull. It is sometimes termed the median or mid-sagittal plane and divides the body into right and left halves. (5)

> Coronal planes: these planes are named after the coronal suture of the skull. They are sometimes termed frontal planes and they are any plane which divides the body into front (anterior) and back (posterior) portions. Coronal planes are perpendicular to the sagittal plane. (6)

> Transverse planes: these planes are perpendicular to the sagittal and coronal planes. They are sometimes called horizontal or axial planes and pass through the body in a horizontal or transverse directions dividing the body into upper (superior) and lower (inferior) sections. (7)

> Oblique planes: these planes are those which do not pass through the body parallel to the sagittal, coronal, or transverse planes. (8)

Anatomical Position: in order to facilitate a common way to refer to all parts of the body, all comers must share the same frame of reference. This is accomplished by considering the body in a specific pose called the anatomical position. In this pose the body is erect, the head faces forward, the feet are together facing forward and the upper limbs face forward (with palms facing forward and thumbs pointing out, away from the body). (9)

Superficial: this refers to structures which are closer to the body's surface than are deeper structures. As an example, the thyroid gland is superficial to the trachea.

Deep: this refers to structures which are farther from the body's surface than are superficial structures. As an example, the trachea is deep to the thyroid gland.

Superior: this refers to structures which are more toward the top of the head. Sometimes the term cranial is used instead. As an example, the eyes are superior to the nose.

Inferior: this refers to structures which are more toward the feet. Sometimes the term caudal is used instead. As an example, the nose is inferior to the eyes.

Anterior: this refers to structures which are toward the front of the body. Sometimes the term ventral is used instead. As an example, the sternum is anterior to the spinal column.

Posterior: this refers to structures which are toward the back of the body. Sometimes the term dorsal is used instead. As an example, the spinal column is posterior to the sternum.

Medial: this refers to structures which are toward the midline of the body. As an example, the middle ear is medial to the outer ear.

Lateral: this refers to structures which are toward the outside (farther from the midline) aspect of the body. As an example, the outer ear is lateral to the middle ear.

Median: this refers to structures which lie on the midline of the body. Examples are the nose, trachea, and sternum.

Proximal: this refers to locations along linear structures which are closer to the structure's origin (or are "upstream" on the structure) than another location. As an example, the ascending colon is proximal to the transverse colon.

Distal: this refers to locations along linear structures which are farther from the structure's origin (or are "downstream" on the structure) than another location. As an example, the descending colon is distal to the transverse colon.

Abduct: this refers to the movement of a structure of the body away from the midline or away from another part.

Adduct: this refers to the movement of a structure of the body toward the midline or toward another part.

Flexion: to decrease the angle between two adjacent structures.

Extension: to increase the angle between two adjacent structures.

Sources Cited:

1-4. Brzezinski, et al. Laboratory and Study Guide for Head and Neck Anatomy: Dissection of the Head and Neck. Ann Arbor, MI. 2013

5-9. Medical Gross Anatomy Learning Modules - Anatomical Orientation. 2000. http://www.med.umich.edu/lrc/coursepages/m1/anatomy2010/html/courseinfo/module_index.html

Scalp, Cranial Cavity, and Meninges

Introduction

This chapter will cover the internal and external aspects of the human skull. In particular, it will examine the scalp which covers the skull externally, the cranial vault or internal cavity of the skull, the meninges which line the brain and the skull, the brain itself, the ventricular system which produces cerebrospinal fluid, the arterial supply to the brain, and the venous drainage of the brain.

Bones of the Skull

The human skull is a complex bony structure. Collectively, there are 22 bones which work together to form the skull. Of these 22 bones, 8 are cranial bones and 14 are facial bones.
- Cranial Bones:
    - Frontal
    - Occipital
    - Ethmoid
    - Sphenoid
    - Parietal (2 total: one on each side of the skull)
    - Temporal (2 total: one on each side of the skull)
- Facial Bones:
    - Mandible
    - Vomer
    - Maxilla (2 total: one on each side of the face)
    - Lacrimal (2 total: one on each side of the face)
    - Palatine (2 total: one on each side of the face)
    - Zygomatic (2 total: one on each side of the face)
    - Nasal (2 total: one on each side of the face)
    - Inferior Nasal Conchae (2 total: one on each side of the face)

The student should find these bones in an atlas of human anatomy and commit their locations to memory. You will be exposed to all of these bones individually throughout any head and neck anatomy course and you should begin to understand them at an early point in your studies.

Bony Sutures

Sutures form where the various bones of the skull fuse together. Since the skull is composed of many bones, there are many sites of bony fusion (technically, a special type of joint).

Early in life (both before and immediately after birth) the bones of the skull must not be fused in order to allow for growth of the brain. As the brain develops, the volume of the skull must expand in order to accommodate the growing central nervous system. The "open" areas between the bones of the skull before fusion occurs are called fontanelles. There are many named fontanelles, but the two most important are the anterior fontanelle and the posterior fontanelle. The <u>anterior fontanelle</u> is the open region between the frontal bone and the parietal bones and it typically closes between 9 and 18 months of age. The <u>posterior fontanelle</u> is the open region between the parietal bones and the occipital bone and it typically closes before the newborn reaches 2 months of age.

Eventually, the rapid growth of the brain slows and the bones of the skull come together and permanently fuse. If the sutures close too early the brain will not have room to expand as it develops. Early closure is clinically referred to as <u>craniosynostosis</u> and must be treated surgically.

- Key Sutures:
    - o The coronal suture lies between the frontal bone and parietal bones.
    - o The sagittal suture lies between the parietal bones.
- Other Sutures:
    - o Lambdoidal
    - o Squamosal
    - o Sphenosquamosal
    - o Zygomaticomaxillary
    - o Zygomaticofrontal
    - o Frontonasal

An important region where the frontal, parietal, sphenoid, and temporal bones meet is called the pterion. It is a weak area and prone to fracture. Immediately deep to the pterion is the middle meningeal artery which supplies the meningeal linings of the brain. The middle meningeal artery is found between the dura mater and the bony skull. It carves a path through the bone of the calvarium (top of the bony skull) after it enters the skull via the foramen spinosum. It originates from the maxillary artery in the midface.

If the pterion is fractured, the middle meningeal artery may be compromised allowing blood to accumulate between the dura mater and the bony skull. This extravasation of blood is known as an epidural hematoma and will be discussed later in this lesson.

<u>Taking Apart The Skull</u>

The uppermost, or top of the skull is called the skull cap, calvaria, or the calvarium. The anterior portion is formed by the frontal bone. Most of the bulk of the skull cap is formed by the parietal bones. Only a small, posterior portion of the skull cap is formed by the occipital bone.

If one were to look at the internal aspect of the skull cap one would notice that the grooves for the middle meningeal artery are visible as they carve their way through the bone bilaterally. The middle meningeal artery serves both the meninges and the skull cap.

The internal skull base can be divided into three regions: the anterior, middle, and posterior cranial fossae. These regions are unique and contain specific anatomic structures which will be discussed in further detail.

- The anterior cranial fossa lies directly above the orbital cavities and nasal cavities. In the median aspect of the anterior cranial fossa one finds the cribriform plate with its foramina. These small openings allow passage of olfactory nerve (CN I) fibers as they supply the superior aspect of the nasal cavity with the sense of smell. The anterior portion of the anterior cranial fossa is formed by the frontal bone. The posterior portion is formed by the lesser wing of the sphenoid bone.

- The middle cranial fossa is formed anteriorly by the greater wing of the sphenoid bone and by the petrous ridge of the temporal bone posteriorly. It houses the foramen rotundum (containing V2 trigeminal nerve fibers), the foramen ovale (containing V3 trigeminal nerve fibers), and the foramen spinosum (which allows passage for the middle meningeal artery). The hypophyseal fossa also resides within the middle cranial fossa and contains the pituitary gland. The hypophyseal fossa is bounded by the tuberculum and dorsum sellae. As is true in other areas of the skull, the prevalence of multiple foramina in the middle cranial fossa weakens the surrounding bone and heightens the possibility of fractures in trauma.

- The posterior cranial fossa is formed primarily by the occipital bone and allows for exit of the spinal cord from the skull via the foramen magnum. The foramen magnum is also the opening by which the vertebral arteries gain access to the inner aspect of the skull. It is important to note that the posterior cranial fossa houses the internal acoustic meatus (containing CN VII and CN VIII fibers), the jugular foramen (containing CN IX, X, and XI fibers along with the internal jugular vein), and the hypoglossal canal which allows the exit of the hypoglossal nerve (CN XII) on its way to efferently innervate the tongue.

Skull Fractures

Fractures of the skull base are not uncommon in the context of trauma given the weakness of the area (due to sutures and foramina).

Fractures of the anterior cranial fossa may allow the egress of blood or other fluids from the cranial vault into the face. Since the anterior cranial fossa lies directly superior to the orbital and nasal cavities, extravasation of blood may find its way into the orbital or nasal cavities following fracture of the anterior fossa floor.

Leakage of fluids from the nose is referred to as rhinorrea. Leakage of fluids into the orbital space may give rise to the panda bear sign as the skin at the external aspect of the orbit becomes ecchymotic (bruised).

Fractures of the middle cranial fossa may allow the egress of blood or other fluids from the cranial vault into the soft tissues behind the ear, or into the ear and nasal cavities themselves.

Leakage of fluids from the ear is referred to as otorrhea. Leakage of fluids from the middle ear space into the nasal cavity is accomplished via the auditory tube passing between the middle ear and the nasopharynx (region directly posterior to the nasal cavity).

The External Skull Base

The serious head and neck student should study the inferior and external surface of the skull base. This can be accomplished via the use of an actual skull and/or an anatomy atlas. The various bony contributions of the skull should be identified and reviewed.

There are many openings in the skull base. These openings are formed when bone embryologically forms around developing arteries, veins, and nerves. In an atlas or on a specimen, note specifically the foramen spinosum (transmitting the middle meningeal artery), carotid canal (transmitting the internal carotid artery), and the jugular foramen (transmitting the internal jugular vein as well as cranial nerves IX, X, and XI).

The foramen lacerum is not as large as most anatomy atlases show it. It is also not as large in the living human as dried anatomic skulls show it. When skulls are dried and bleached for anatomic study the foramen lacerum typically enlarges as an artifact of preservation. However, the foramen lacerum does contain various structures, and functionally it allows the transmission of petrosal nerves and smaller venous structures into and out of the skull.

The hypoglossal canal allows the transmission of the hypoglossal nerve (CN XII) out of the cranial vault and is located lateral to the occipital condyle which articulates with the first cervical vertebra.

Finally, the foramen magnum resides entirely within the occipital bone and allows the transmission of the spinal cord and vertebral blood vessels out of and into the skull, respectively. As an aside, the foramen magnum also allows entrance of the spinal accessory nerve (CN XI) into the skull since this cranial nerve arises from the inferior brainstem and superior spinal cord. The spinal accessory nerve will subsequently leave the skull via the jugular foramen with CN IX and CN X.

The Internal Skull Base

The serious head and neck student should also study the internal surface of the skull base. Again, this can be accomplished via the use of an actual skull and/or an anatomy atlas.

Certain features of the various foramina discussed in the previous sections titled "The External Skull Base" and "Taking Apart The Skull" can also be seen on the internal aspect of the skull. These foramina pass from internal to external.

In addition to the aforementioned foramina, one can see various additional foramina and bony openings on the internal aspect of the skull which are not visible from an external visualization.

Note that one can here appreciate the optic canal (transmitting CN II), the superior orbital fissure (transmitting CN III, IV, and the ophthalmic nerve), foramen rotundum (transmitting the maxillary nerve), and foramen ovale (transmitting the mandibular nerve).

The internal acoustic meatus transmits CN VII and VIII into the inner ear.

Scalp

The scalp refers to the covering of skin and tissues which lie superior to the calvarium.

The scalp can be subdivided into five primary layers. The first and most superficial layer is the skin. The skin is composed of the deeper dermis and more superficial epidermis. The second layer is a connective tissue layer which is dense and highly vascularized. The third layer is an aponeurotic layer and contains the occipitofrontalis muscle bellies. The fourth layer is another connective tissue layer, but is loose. This layer allows for the spread of infection beneath the superficial layers of the scalp. The fifth, deepest, and final layer of the scalp is the pericranial layer which is tightly adherent to the calvarium.

In general, the scalp is highly vascularized and is afferently innervated by branches of the trigeminal nerve.

The Meninges

There are three meningeal layers which protect the central nervous system (including the brain and spinal cord). These three layers are the pia mater, the arachnoid mater, and the dura mater.

The pia mater is very thin, and is tightly adherent to the brain surface itself.

The arachnoid mater is "spider-web-like", and lies between the pia mater and the dura mater. Cerebrospinal fluid (which is formed via the choroid plexuses in the ventricular system) resides between the pia and arachnoid mater in the subarachnoid space.

The cranial dura mater is the most superficial layer of the meningeal linings. It is very tough and lies adherent to the periosteal lining of the bony skull. It is continuous through the foramen magnum with the spinal dura mater. The cranial dura mater becomes specialized as it invaginates between regions of the brain. If invagination occurs, a space may be formed between the dura mater and the periosteal lining. This space is a dural venous sinus. The dural venous sinuses drain blood from the scalp, skull bones (diploic veins) and brain back to the heart. Emissary veins interconnect scalp and diploic veins with the dural venous sinuses and the vertebral venous plexus of the spinal column. They have a special endothelial lining, but unlike veins, they contain no valves. (1, p. 22)

If no space is formed, the invaginating layers of dura mater adhere to each other forming various dural partitions. The falx cerebri separates the left and right parts of the cerebrum. The falx cerebelli separates the left and right parts of the cerebellum. The tentorium cerebelli separates the cerebrum from the cerebellum.

The meninges and the scalp are served by the trigeminal (and, to a lesser extent, cervical) nerves.

Interestingly, the brain itself is relatively insensitive to pain and sensation. Clinically, therefore, most headaches are vascular or dural in nature.

Hematomas

The brain and its support structures are highly vascularized. Arteries supply them and veins take deoxygenated blood away from them. Normally, blood stays in the arterial and venous systems. Sometimes, pathologically, blood may escape the vasculature and cause serious clinical problems.

Epidural hematomas are typically the result of a ruptured middle meningeal artery with subsequent bleeding into the space between the dura mater and the bony skull. The collection of blood which forms within that space is "convex" in shape. The center of the epidural hematoma is essentially the area where the extravasated blood has pushed the dura mater away from the periosteal lining toward the brain's surface.

Epidural hematomas give rise to various signs and symptoms (as cranial nerves are impacted from the mass affect of the collection of blood), but a fixed and dilated pupil may be one of the most readily observed signs as the third cranial nerve is compromised.

In contrast, subdural hematomas are caused when bridging veins are shorn. Blood accumulates below the dura mater and spreads out over the surface of the brain giving a "concave" appearance on radiographic imaging.

Lobes of the Brain

The brain is a highly complex organ and is examined in depth in any of a number of neuroanatomy and neuroscience textbooks. It will not be studied in detail in this resource. However, a few basic points of neuroanatomy are important as one visualizes the undissected brain.

Anteriorly one finds the frontal lobe.

Posterior to the central sulcus (and the frontal lobe) one finds the parietal lobes.

Inferior to the parietooccipital sulcus one finds the occipital lobe.

Inferior to the cerebrum is the cerebellum (posteriorly) and the brainstem (anteriorly).

The brainstem is an important structure inferior to the cerebrum. It is formed by the midbrain, pons, and medulla oblongata. It is the site of origination of ten of the twelve cranial nerves and controls various functions, many of which the body performs "unconsciously". The various cranial nerves will be explained in detail elsewhere, but one should know that they arise from the brainstem. CN III and IV arise from the midbrain, CN V-VIII arise from the pons, and CN IX-XII arise from the medulla. Cranial nerves I and II technically arise from the forebrain.

The thalamus and hypothalamus as well as the ventricular system are central structures within the central nervous system. The pituitary gland is immediately inferior to the hypothalamus. The basic surface features of the brain may be summarized as follows (2, p. 25):

- Forebrain
    - o Telencephalon
        - ▪ Cerebral Hemispheres (contains the lateral ventricles)
            - Longitudinal Fissure (a.k.a. superior sagittal sulcus)
            - Sulci
                - o Central
                - o Parietooccipital
                - o Lateral (a.k.a. lateral fissure)
            - Lobes
                - o Frontal
                - o Parietal
                - o Temporal
                - o Occipital
    - o Diencephalon (contains the 3rd ventricle; origin of CN II)
        - Pituitary Stalk
- Midbrain (mesencephalon) (contains the cerebral aqueduct; origin of CN III & IV)
    - o Cerebral Peduncles

- <u>Hindbrain</u> (rhombencephalon) (contains the 4th ventricle)
  - o Pons (Origin of CN V, VI, VII & VIII)
  - o Medulla Oblongata (Origin of CN IX, X, XI & XII)
    - ▪ Pyramids
    - ▪ Olives
  - o Cerebellum
    - ▪ Hemispheres

Ventricular System

Located centrally in the brain parenchyma we find the ventricular system. The lateral ventricles are found in the telencephalon, while the third ventricle is found in the diencephalon and the fourth ventricle is found in the brainstem.

The ventricular system is vitally important since it is the site of cerebrospinal fluid synthesis. Cerebrospinal fluid is formed via the choroid plexuses (specialized tissue found in all of the ventricles) and exits the ventricular system by means of small apertures (lateral and median) in the fourth ventricle whereby it enters the subarachnoid space.

The cerebrospinal fluid then bathes the central nervous system's exterior within the subarachnoid space.

The cerebrospinal fluid eventually drains back into dural venous sinuses via arachnoid granulations and then ultimately into the systemic venous circulation. Since cerebrospinal fluid is continuously being formed it must also continuously leave the subarachnoid space so that pressure differentials remain constant within the cranial vault.

Arachnoid granulations are specializations of the arachnoid mater which project into the dural venous sinuses in order to return cerebrospinal fluid to the vascular system. These granulations carve granular fovea on the inner surface of the skull cap. The dural venous sinuses eventually drain into larger veins (such as the internal jugular vein) returning blood to the heart. In this way cerebrospinal fluid may be produced in the ventricles, find its way to the subarachnoid space, and ultimately be drained into the systemic circulation so that a constant pressure is maintained in the subarachnoid space.

<u>Hydrocephalus</u> results when cerebrospinal fluid does not exit the subarachnoid space at an equivalent pace to its production in the ventricles. In other words, there is an increased quantity of cerebrospinal fluid in the subarachnoid space due to either overproduction or obstructed drainage. An increased quantity of cerebrospinal fluid increases the pressure in the cranial vault leading to potential neurological sequela.

Arterial Supply to the Brain

The cranial vault and its contents are supplied by the vertebral arteries (posteriorly) and the internal carotid arteries (anteriorly).

The vertebral arteries arise from the subclavian arteries in the thorax bilaterally. They then travel toward the head through the transverse foramina of vertebrae C6-C1 before entering the cranial vault via the foramen magnum.

The internal carotid arteries split off from the common carotid arteries near the level of the hyoid bone and travel toward the head before entering the cranial vault via the carotid canals. There are no branches from the internal carotid arteries in the neck, and it is the primary vascular supply to the brain.

In the cranial vault the vertebral arteries anastomose with the internal carotid arteries forming the Circle of Willis. This arrangement ensures that the brain receives sufficient oxygenation even in the event of compromised blood flow in one of the contributing arteries. The Circle of Willis is formed by the posterior cerebral, posterior communicating, middle cerebral, anterior cerebral, and anterior communicating arteries.

It should be noted that the vertebral arteries come together to form the basilar artery. The basilar then anastomoses with the internal carotid arteries on the anterior surface of the brainstem. The basilar artery gives rise to the posterior cerebral arteries. These are the primary arteries which supply the posteroinferior portion of the cerebrum.

The internal carotid arteries give rise to the middle and anterior cerebral arteries. These are the primary arteries which supply the anterosuperior portion of the cerebrum.

Communicating arteries complete the Circle of Willis and allow for complete anastomosis.

It should be noted that the pituitary gland passes inferiorly through the Circle of Willis.

As a historical side note, Thomas Willis was an English physician who studied the nervous system. He was also an Oxford professor and wrote *Cerebri Anatome, Cui Accessit Nervorum Descriptio Et Usus* (1664; "Anatomy of the Brain, with a Description of the Nerves and Their Function") where he first described the anastomoses of the blood supply to the brain.

The Circle of Willis is commonly taught as described in this chapter, but you should understand that its anatomic arrangement is highly variable from body to body. It is found as described here approximately 20% of the time.

Regardless of the specific arrangement of the Circle of Willis, the take home point is that anastomoses of blood vessels (from the vertebral and internal carotid arteries) occurs at the base of the brain in order to ensure adequate oxygenation to neural tissues.

A subarachnoid hemorrhage occurs as blood enters the subarachnoid space. This typically occurs when an aneurysm found within the Circle of Willis ruptures.

The anterior circulation of the cerebrum is supplied by the internal carotid arteries. The anterior circulation is distributed via the anterior and middle cerebral arteries.

The posterior circulation of the cerebrum (and cerebellum) is supplied by the vertebral arteries. The brainstem is also largely supplied by the vertebral arteries. The posterior circulation is distributed via the posterior cerebral (and cerebellar) arteries.

Specific regions of the brain are supplied by specific cerebral arteries. You should take the time to memorize the general regions supplied by the specific arteries.

Venous Drainage From the Brain

Scalp veins, bridging veins, emissary veins, and diploic veins drain superficial structures into the dural venous sinuses. Veins on the surface of the brain also drain into the dural venous sinuses. The dural venous sinuses cut corresponding grooves on the endocranial surface of the skull.

The superior sagittal sinus and inferior sagittal sinus are found at the top and bottom of the falx cerebri (respectively). They are connected via the straight sinus and ultimately drain into the confluence of sinuses at the posterior aspect of the cranial vault. An occipital sinus also drains into the confluence from below.

The right and left transverse sinuses arise from the confluence and pass anterolaterally until they dive inferiorly as the sigmoid sinuses. These sigmoid sinuses also receive smaller petrosal branches which serve to drain blood from the anteriorly placed cavernous sinus. The blood within the sigmoid sinuses passes inferiorly out of the cranial vault via the jugular foramina. As the sigmoids pass through the jugular foramina they are renamed the internal jugular veins. The internal jugular veins pass inferiorly through the neck until they ultimately reach the right side of the heart and lungs for oxygenation.

It is clinically important to note that various veins of the upper and midface region pass posteriorly through the orbit and interconnect with the dural venous sinuses (via the cavernous sinus). This arrangement is potentially dangerous if infectious pathogens find their way into the sinus spaces. For this reason the clinician should aggressively treat facial lacerations and infections.

The cavernous sinuses lie on either side of the body of the sphenoid bone around the pituitary gland in the middle cranial fossa. Various cranial nerves exit the cranial vault by passing through the cavernous sinus space. These nerves include CN III, IV, V-1 and V-2, as well as VI (abducens nerve). The internal carotid artery also passes through the cavernous sinus space.

It is important to note that most structures passing through the sinus pass through along its lateral walls. The internal carotid artery and abducens nerve, however, pass through the center of the cavernous sinus.

If any infection sets up shop in the cavernous sinus space (from an infected facial laceration, for example), the blood in the sinus may clot (thrombose) and an abscess may form. This is clinically significant because the internal carotid artery may be compromised (leading to a hemorrhagic stroke) if the infection erodes through its walls. The abducens nerve may also be compromised leading to the inability to abduct the eye on the affected side (given the role of CN VI). Structures along the lateral wall of the cavernous sinus space are largely unaffected in such circumstances. Infections of the cavernous sinus can be treated with antibiotics, but abscesses sometimes can be difficult to eradicate without physical evacuation of the infection.

Sources Cited:

1-2. Brzezinski, et al. Laboratory and Study Guide for Head and Neck Anatomy: Dissection of the Head and Neck. Ann Arbor, MI. 2013

Laboratory Approach

☐1. Examine the soft tissue (scalp) which covers the calvarium. Distinguish the five layers of the scalp and note individual relationships between adjacent layers. The scalp may be removed from the skull.

☐2. Examine the calvarium or skull cap. Look for sutures, foramina and any grooves from neurovasculature.

☐3. Examine the internal and external skull base. Identify bony foramina and determine which neurovascular structures traverse the various openings.

☐4. Examine the cranial meninges and distinguish their three layers. Identify the specializations of the dura mater which lie between certain regions of the brain tissue.

☐5. Examine the dural venous sinuses and be able to describe the flow of blood through them.

☐6. Examine the bones of the skull on a dry specimen. Identify the major sutures and openings which are visible.

☐7. Examine the gross features of the brain including the major lobes, sulci, and grooves.

☐8. Examine the brainstem and identify the cranial nerves which arise from the brainstem. Be sure to understand the function(s) of the nerves and their exit openings within the skull.

☐9. Examine the arterial supply to the brain via the internal carotid arteries and the vertebral arteries. Describe how the Circle of Willis is formed and its importance.

Key Regional Structures

Cranial meninges
  Pia
  Arachnoid
    subarachnoid space
    arachnoid granulations
    granular foveae (carved into bone)
  Dura
    periosteal dura
    meningeal dura
      dural septa
          falx cerebri
        tentorium cerebelli
            tentorial notch
        falx cerebelli
        diaphragma sellae
      dural venous sinuses
        superior sagittal
        inferior sagittal
        confluens
        straight
        transverse
        occipital
        sigmoid
        cavernous
        ant. & post. intercavernous
        sphenoparietal
        sup. & inf. petrosal
        basilar (plexus)
Internal jugular vein
Vertebral venous plexuses
Emissary veins
Hypophysis (pituitary gland)
Vertebral arteries
    Ant. & post. spinal arteries
    Post. inf. cerebellar arteries
Internal carotid artery
    Middle cerebral artery
    Basilar artery
      Sup. cerebellar branch
      Ant. inf. cerebellar branch
Arterial Circle of Willis
    posterior cerebral arteries
    posterior communicating arteries
    anterior cerebral arteries
    anterior communicating arteries
Cranial Nerves (I-XII)
Cerebral Lobes and Cerebellum
Brainstem
Scalp

ANTERIOR, MIDDLE AND POSTERIOR CRANIAL FOSSA
FORAMEN MAGNUM
JUGULAR FORAMEN
SUPERIOR ORBITAL FISSURE
INFERIOR ORBITAL FISURE
FORAMEN ROTUNDUM
FORAMEN OVALE
CLIVUS
GREATER and LESSER WING of SPHENOID BONE
STYLOID PROCESS
MASTOID PROCESS
PHARYNGEAL TUBERCLE
PETROUS PORTION of TEMPORAL BONE
HYPOPHYSEAL FOSSA
ANTERIOR CLINOID PROCESSES
POSTERIOR CLINOID PROCESSES
EXTERNAL OPENING of CAROTID CANAL
HYPOGLOSSAL CANAL
INTERNAL ACOUSTIC MEATUS
EXTERNAL ACOUSTIC MEATUS
FORAMEN LACERUM

BONES OF THE CRANIAL VAULT (8):
FRONTAL
OCCIPITAL
ETHMOID
SPHENOID
PARIETAL (2)
TEMPORAL (2)

BONES OF THE FACIAL SKELETON (14):
LACRIMAL (2)
PALATINE (2)
ZYGOMATIC (2)
NASAL (2)
MAXILLA (2)
INFERIOR NASAL CONCHAE (2)
MANDIBLE
VOMER

SUTURES:
CORONAL
SAGITTAL
LAMBDOIDAL
SQUAMOSAL
SPHENOSQUAMOSAL
ZYGOMATICOMAXILLARY
ZYGOMATICOFRONTAL
FRONTONASAL

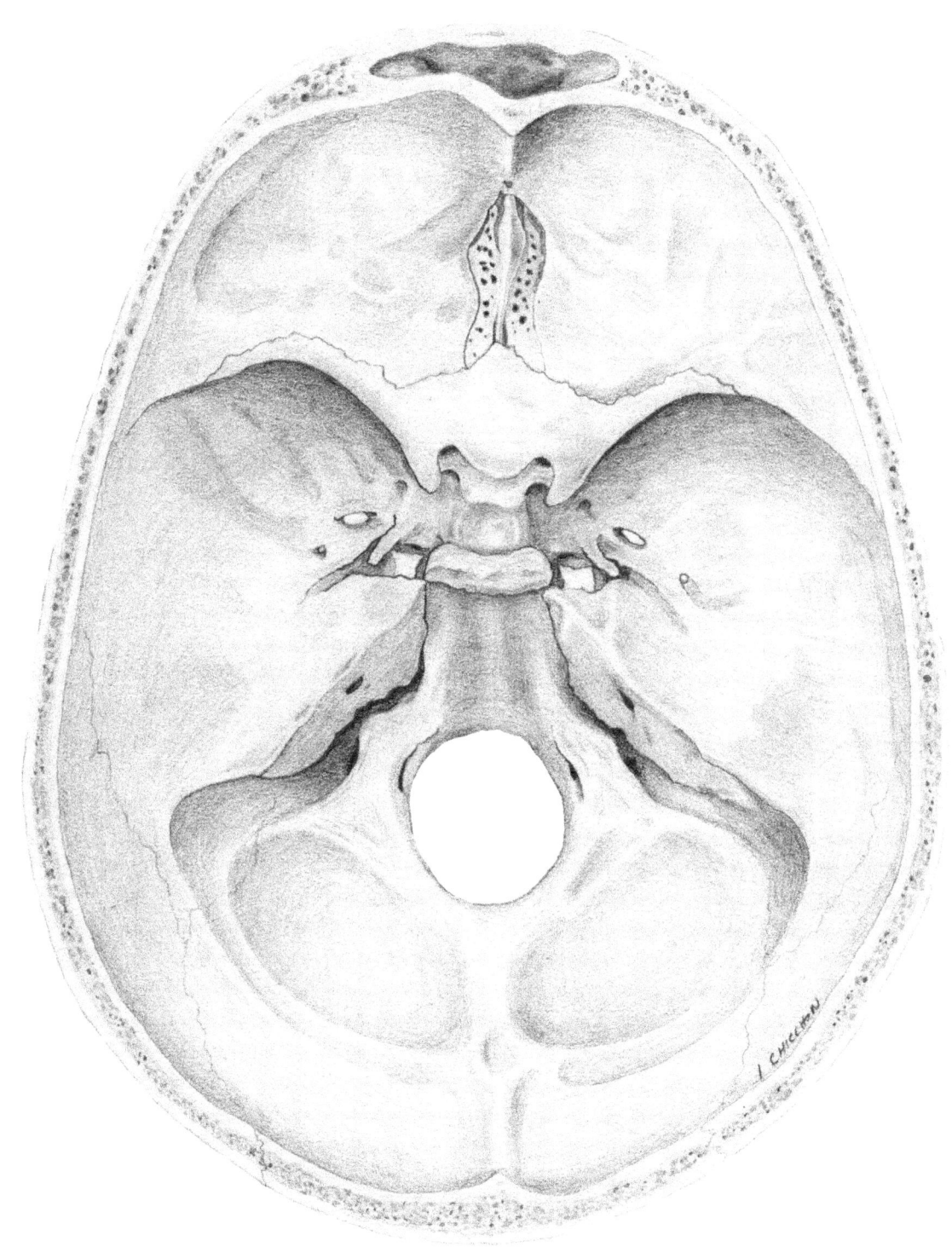

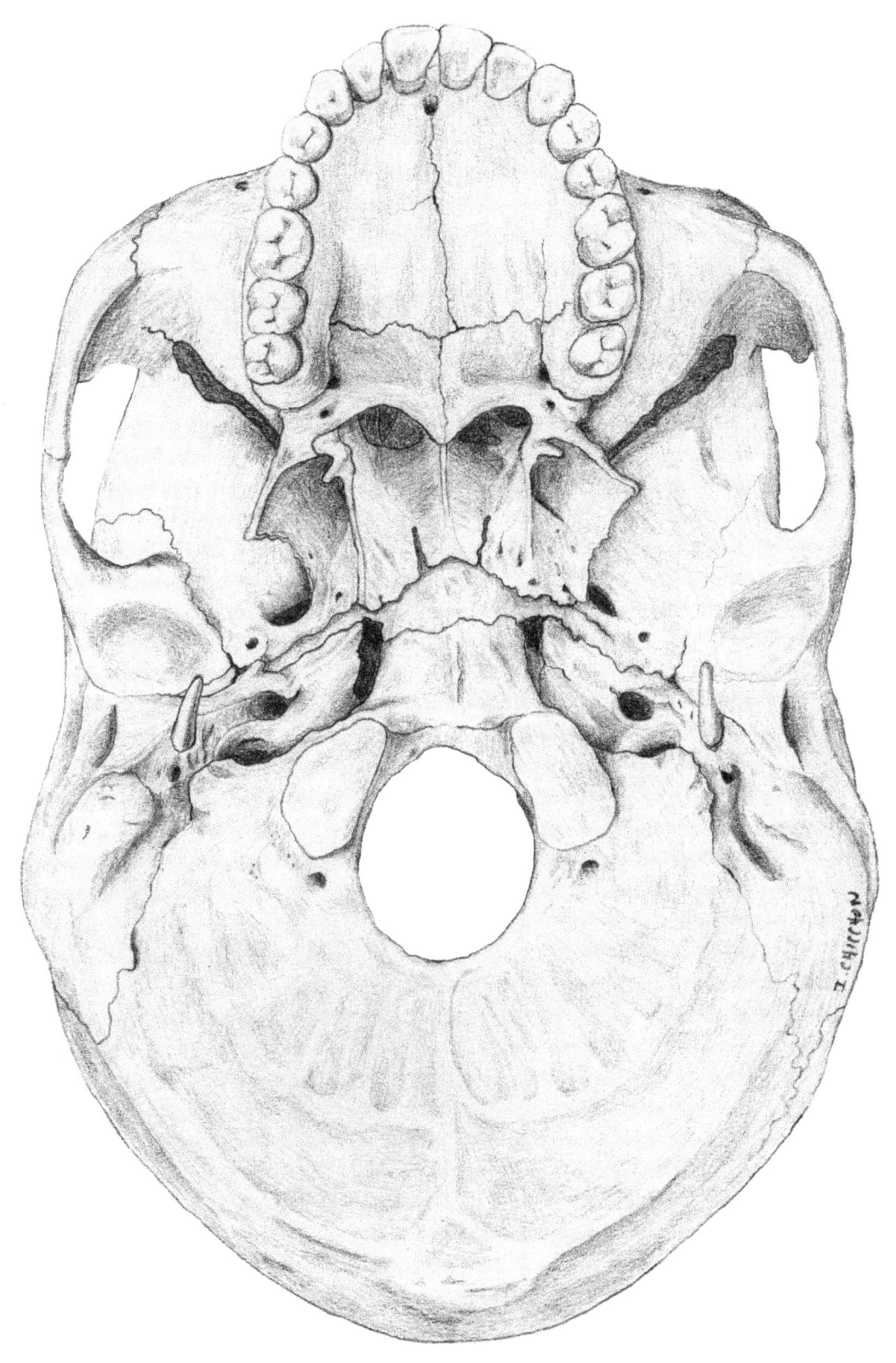

Anterior Neck

Introduction

This chapter will introduce the neck with specific attention given to the anterior neck. The neck is a very important structure anatomically and clinically. While its most obvious function may be to provide support for the head, it also serves to provide an important connection between the head and the thorax. Neurovascular structures pass back and forth between the head and the thorax via the neck. Other important structures, including the trachea and esophagus, also pass between the head and the thorax by means of the neck.

In order to facilitate communication between clinicians and in order to describe the anatomy accurately, the neck can be divided into anterior and posterior regions. These geographic regions may be further subdivided into complex fascial spaces and compartments.

Neck Divisions

The anterior neck is essentially that portion of the neck anterior to the spinal column. It contains a central visceral compartment, two neurovascular bundles (one on each side of the visceral compartment), and a relatively thin layer of musculature. The posterior neck contains the vertebral column, the spinal cord, the trapezius and levator scapulae muscles, and the deep musculature of the neck which surrounds and supports the vertebral column. (1, p. 33)

The anterior and posterior neck may then be further subdivided into complex fascial spaces. The layers of fascia which surround various structures in the neck serve to isolate and compartmentalize these structures. The fascia in the neck is referred to as cervical fascia.

Fascia is found throughout the body surrounding bones, muscles, organs, and neurovasculature. It envelops these structures like a sheet. It is composed of connective tissue and serves as mechanistic support for the body's organs and structures.

Clinically, fascial spaces or compartments are important because the regions between these compartments permit the movement of fluids and pathogens. Infection, for example, may travel from the head to the thorax along these fascial planes. Similarly, infection may develop within a fascial compartment. Such compartmentalization isolates the pathogen and may impede proper healing. In cases such as these the clinician must surgically open the compartment and drain the infectious material. (2, p. 33)

The Skeleton of the Neck

The neck functions to support the head. It does this by means of direct bony articulation (i.e. the spinal column is directly connected to the occipital bone of the external skull base). It also does this by means of muscular attachments between the skull and spinal column.

The spinal column runs the entire length of the back from the skull superiorly to the hip bones inferiorly. The spinal column of the neck is formed from seven vertebral bones. These seven bones are the seven most superior vertebral bones in the spinal column and are referred to as cervical vertebrae.

Cervical vertebra number seven (a.k.a. C7) is the inferior-most cervical vertebra. Its spinous process can be palpated as the patient flexes his or her neck forward.

Within the vertebral bones resides the spinal cord.

Immediately anterior to the spinal column (and its vertebral bones) are the hyoid bone, larynx, and trachea. These structures are accessory skeletal structures and constitute a combination of both bony and soft tissues. The hyoid bone is anterior to the third cervical vertebra and is the attachment point for strap and tongue muscles. It is connected to the skull by means of the stylohyoid ligament. It is connected to the larynx via the thyrohyoid membrane. The larynx is composed of the cricoid cartilage and the thyroid cartilage. It, in turn, is connected to the trachea which resides immediately inferior to it. These anterior neck structures will be examined in further detail later in this book. At this point, you should begin to familiarize yourself with their location in the neck, recognizing that other soft tissue structures will be described in relationship to them.

Nerves Arising from the Neck

The portion of the spinal cord traversing the neck gives rise to eight cervical nerves (C1 – C8) which afferently and efferently serve neck and upper limb structures. They have both ventral (anterior) and dorsal (posterior) rami which serve the anterior and posterior portions of the head and neck (respectively).

Recall that afferent nerves bring sensory information from the periphery back to the central nervous system while efferent nerves deliver motor signals from the central nervous system to effector muscles of the periphery.

The cervical plexus of nerves is formed from the ventral primary rami of spinal nerves C1 to C4. The brachial plexus of nerves is formed from the ventral primary rami of spinal nerves C5 – C8 as well as T1 (the first spinal nerve arising from the superior portion of the thoracic spinal cord).

The cervical plexus of nerves afferently innervates the cutaneous tissues of the anterior neck. The cervical plexus of nerves also efferently innervates the strap muscles of the anterior neck (via the ansa cervicalis).

While most of the tasks of cervical spinal nerves pertain to the neck, some do not. The phrenic nerve (C3, 4, 5) arises from cervical spinal nerves and innervates the diaphragm and allows for respiration.

As an aside, the face is innervated afferently by the trigeminal nerve (V1, V2, and V3 fibers) and not cervical spinal nerves. The only exception to this rule is the area of tissue immediately overlying the angle of the mandible which is afferently innervated by C2, C3 fibers (via the great auricular nerve). It is the anterior and posterior necks which are afferently innervated primarily by C2, C3, and C4 fibers.

Triangles of the Neck

To facilitated communication between clinicians and to accurately describe the anatomy, the neck can be divided into triangles. Various structures of the anterior and posterior neck may be described as residing within certain triangles.

There are two "major" triangles. The major triangles are the anterior and posterior triangles.

The anterior triangle contains the area bounded medially by the midline, laterally by the anterior border of the sternocleidomastoid muscle, and superiorly by the lower border of the mandible.

The posterior triangle contains the area bounded anteriorly by the sternocleidomastoid muscle, posteriorly by the trapezius muscle, and inferiorly by the clavicle.

Both the anterior and posterior triangles can be further subdivided into additional smaller triangles.

Anterior triangle subdivisions:
- Muscular triangle (boundaries):
    o medial: midline
    o superolateral: superior belly of the omohyoid muscle
    o inferolateral: sternocleidomastoid muscle
- Submandibular triangle (boundaries)
    o anterior: anterior belly of the digastric muscle
    o posterior: posterior belly of the digastric muscle
    o superior: lower border of the mandible
- Submental triangle (boundaries)
    o lateral: both digastric muscles (anterior bellies)
    o inferior: hyoid bone
- Carotid triangle (boundaries)
    o lateral: sternocleidomastoid muscle
    o superior: posterior belly of the digastric muscle
    o anterior: superior belly of the omohyoid muscle

Posterior triangle subdivisions:
- Subclavian/Omoclavicular triangle
    o superior: inferior belly of omohyoid muscle
    o anterior: sternocleidomastoid muscle
    o inferior: clavicle
- Occipital triangle
    o anterior: sternocleidomastoid muscle
    o posterior: trapezius muscle
    o inferior: omohyoid muscle

Fascial Layers of the Neck

Every structure in the neck is individually covered with a thin layer of fascia.

In addition to thin layers of fascia surrounding every individual structure, thicker layers of fascia invest specific muscular, neurovascular, and visceral groups.

The superficial layer of deep cervical fascia invests the sternocleidomastoid muscles and the trapezius muscles. It forms a complete sheath around the entire neck.

Deep to the superficial layer of deep cervical fascia lies the muscular fascia (a.k.a. the infrahyoid fascia). The muscular fascia invests the strap muscles (a.k.a. infrahyoid muscles).

Deep to the muscular fascia lies the visceral fascia which surrounds the thyroid gland, esophagus, and trachea. This visceral fascia is subdivided anteriorly into the pretracheal fascia and posteriorly into the buccopharyngeal fascia.

Slightly lateral and deep to the visceral fascia lie the carotid sheaths. The carotid sheath fascia surrounds the internal jugular vein, carotid artery, and vagus nerve (CN X) bilaterally.

Finally, the spinal column and deep musculature which supports it are invested by a thick sheet of fascia known as the prevertebral fascia.

Infectious pathogens can readily travel from the head to the thorax via the "highways" created between these fascial compartments. Most importantly, the space immediately anterior to the prevertebral fascia is the most frequently traversed pathway for pathogens traveling between the head and the thorax.

Superficial Anterior Neck: Platysma Muscles

Initially, the skin and subcutaneous tissue are encountered as one approaches the neck superficially. The subcutaneous tissue is sometimes called the "hypodermis" and consists of superficial fascia and adiposity (fat).

Within the subcutaneous tissue lies the platysma muscle. The platysma is efferently innervated by the cervical branch of the facial nerve (CN VII) and is one of the muscles of facial expression.

The platysma originates from fascia overlying the musculature of the pectoralis major and deltoid muscles. It inserts into the skin of the face at the base of the mandible. Its primary action is to depress the angles of the mouth and also to depress the mandible. (3, Muscles of the Head and Neck - Platysma)

Be aware that the platysma is a very thin muscle and is readily dissected away by overzealous dissectors.

The most important nerves which pass through the platysma are the afferent branches of the cervical plexus destined to innervate the overlying cutaneous tissues.

Middle Lateral Anterior Neck: Sternocleidomastoid Muscles

Deep to the platysma are found the sternocleidomastoid muscles (bilaterally).

The sternocleidomastoid muscles originate from the sternum and the clavicle while inserting into the mastoid processes of the temporal bones (thus the muscle's name!).

The sternocleidomastoid muscle is efferently innervated by the spinal accessory nerve (CN XI). It is afferently served by spinal nerves of the cervical plexus (C2, C3 fibers). This is a very unique arrangement since most named nerves are "mixed" (carrying both afferent and efferent fibers). The trapezius muscle, which is invested in the same deep cervical fascia, is similarly innervated.

The sternocleidomastoid muscle turns the chin "up and out" to the opposite side. In other words, it turns the skull from side to side upon the spinal column.

The carotid sheaths (containing the internal jugular vein, common carotid artery, and vagus nerve) are found deep to the sternocleidomastoid muscles, and the afferent branches of the cervical plexus arise at a point (bilaterally) along sternocleidomastoid's posterior border ("Erb's Point") as they travel from deep to superficial (through the platysma) to innervate the overlying cutaneous tissues. Also deep to the sternocleidomastoid muscles are the infrahyoid muscles.

Deep cervical lymph nodes run the length of the carotid sheath in close proximity to the internal jugular vein. The clinician should palpate this nodal group immediately anterior to the sternocleidomastoid muscle. This nodal group ultimately drains the majority of the head and neck.

Middle Medial Anterior Neck: Infrahyoid Muscles

The infrahyoids are named based upon their origins and insertions. They are the sternohyoid muscles, the omohyoid muscles, the sternothyroid muscles, and the thyrohyoid muscles. They are found medial and superficial to the carotid sheaths and deep to the sternocleidomastoid muscles.

The sternohyoid attaches to the sternum and hyoid bone. The omohyoid attaches to the scapula and hyoid bone. The sternothyroid attaches to the sternum and thyroid cartilage of the larynx. The thyrohyoid attaches to the thyroid cartilage of the larynx and hyoid bone.

Medial and deep to the infrahyoids lie the larynx and trachea.

Inferior to the larynx and deep to the sternothyroid muscles lies the thyroid gland. The thyroid gland is superiorly bounded by the attachment of the sternothyroid muscle at the oblique line of the thyroid cartilage (of the larynx).

The infrahyoids are efferently innervated by the ansa cervicalis (from the cervical plexus) along their lateral borders. This is clinically important because the surgeon may access the airway by reflecting the infrahyoids laterally from a midline or medial approach without damaging any nerves.

It should also be noted that the ansa cervicalis is commonly found lying within the fascia of the carotid sheath. Alternatively, the ansa cervicalis may be found passing directly through the sheath itself.

Cervical Plexus

The cervical plexus will now be discussed in greater detail. As an initial overview, the posterior portion of the head and neck are innervated by dorsal primary rami of the cervical nerves. The anterior neck is innervated by ventral primary rami of the cervical nerves

The cervical plexus consists of nerve fibers from ventral C1, C2, C3, and C4 spinal roots.

Ventral C1, C2, and C3 fibers provide efferent innervation to the infrahyoid musculature via the ansa cervicalis.

Ventral and dorsal C1, C2, C3, and C4 fibers provide afferent innervation to the cutaneous structures of the anterior and posterior neck and posterior head (but not the face). They also provide afferent innervation to the musculature of the neck so that the locations of the muscles in three-dimensional space are known by the central nervous system.

C1, C2, C3, and C4 spinal nerves also supply the deep musculature of the neck which supports the spinal column (including the longus colli, longus capitis, rectus capitis anterior, and rectus capitis lateralis muscles).

Specifically, the transverse cervical nerve is derived from ventral C2 and C3 fibers. It serves the skin of the anterior neck.

The great auricular nerve is derived from ventral C2 and C3 fibers. It serves the skin at the angle of the mandible and the skin posterior to the ear and travels with the external jugular vein. It is important to note that the only region of the face not innervated by the trigeminal nerve is the small portion overlying the angle of the mandible which is served by the great auricular nerve. As long as the skin of the face is being referenced, it should be noted that the ophthalmic branch of the trigeminal nerve (V1) innervates the skin of the nasal bridge, upper eyelids, and forehead. The maxillary branch of the trigeminal nerve (V2) innervates the skin of the upper lip to the skin of the lower eyelid. The mandibular branch of the trigeminal nerve (V3) innervates the skin overlying the mandibular base to the lower lip.

The lesser occipital nerve is derived from ventral C2 and C3 fibers. It serves the skin at the base of the skull posterior to the ear.

The supraclavicular nerve has three major branches: the medial, intermediate, and lateral branches. It serves the skin overlying the clavicle and is derived from ventral C3 and C4 fibers. It is of clinical significance to note that the close association of the supraclavicular nerves (C3 and C4) and the phrenic nerves (C3, C4, and C5) results in diaphragmatic pain being referred to the shoulder. (4, Nerves of the Head and Neck - Supraclavicular)

The roots of the cervical plexus arise through the deep musculature of the neck immediately posterior to the anterior scalene muscles. The scalene muscles are accessory muscles of respiration.

Inferior to the emergence of the cervical plexus can be seen the emergence of the brachial plexus and the subclavian artery. The brachial plexus and the subclavian artery pass between the anterior and middle scalene muscles. The brachial plexus arises from within the spinal column while the subclavian artery is passing upwards from the thorax and over the first rib on its way to supply the upper limb.

The subclavian vein is passing from the limb over the first rib on its way back into the thorax after draining the upper limb. This vein runs immediately anterior to the anterior scalene muscle and is an important clinical site for the placement of central lines.

Deep Neck Muscles: Scalenes

The three scalene muscles, the anterior, middle, and posterior, all originate from the transverse processes of cervical vertebrae. The anterior and middle scalene insert onto the first rib. The posterior scalene inserts onto the second rib.

The brachial plexus and subclavian artery pass between the anterior and middle scalenes.

The subclavian vein passes immediately anterior to the anterior scalene muscle.

All neurovasculature discussed here passes over the first rib in order to serve the upper limb.

Thyroid Gland

The thyroid gland wraps around the trachea in the median visceral compartment. It is an important endocrine gland involved in metabolism.

On the posterior surface of the thyroid gland one may observe the parathyroid glands. The parathyroid glands are important endocrine glands involved in calcium management. There may be as few as two parathyroid glands and there may be as many as six parathyroid glands. The parathyroid glands are typically found "toggled" onto the inferior thyroid arteries. While this location is typical, the parathyroid glands may be found anywhere from the level of the thyroid gland to the mediastinal spaces in the thorax.

The thyroid gland is served by the superior and inferior thyroid arteries. The superior thyroid artery arises from the external carotid artery. The inferior thyroid artery arises from the thyrocervical trunk, which in turn arises from the subclavian vessels. Like other endocrine glands, the thyroid gland is highly vascularized.

The carotid sheaths lie lateral to the thyroid gland bilaterally and are deep to the sternocleidomastoid muscles and infrahyoid muscles.

The thyroid gland is supplied by four arteries (originating from the superior and inferior thyroid arteries) and is drained by six veins.

The superior and middle thyroid veins drain directly into the internal jugular vein. The inferior thyroid veins drain into the brachiocephalic veins.

Embryologically the thyroid gland arises from ventral pharyngeal wall tissue at the foramen cecum (tongue base). It descends inferiorly until it is at the level of the cricoid ring and superior trachea. Sometimes a remnant pyramidal lobe remains. There may also be remnant thyroid tissue at any location along the path of descent. As such, midline cysts in the neck of the pediatric patient are most commonly thyroidal tissue in origination.

Various thyroid pathologies may lead to enlargement of the gland. An enlarged thyroid gland is called a goiter and may result from either hyper or hypo functioning of the gland. The most common cause of goiter world-wide is iodine deficiency resulting in hypothyroidism.

Cranial Nerves of the Anterior Neck

Two important cranial nerves are found in the anterior neck. One is the vagus nerve (CN X) which is found within the carotid sheath. The other is the hypoglossal nerve (CN XII) which is found immediately lateral to the carotid sheath as the nerve courses from the skull base, posteriorly, to the tongue base, anteriorly.

The vagus nerve has many roles which will be outlined elsewhere in this book. One role is serving the larynx both afferently and efferently. Another role is providing parasympathetic autonomic innervation to various organs of the thorax and abdomen.

The hypoglossal nerve has only one role. That role is to provide efferent innervation to the tongue musculature. It is important to note that the superior fibers of the ansa cervicalis appear to arise from the hypoglossal nerve. This appearance is deceiving. The fibers of the ansa cervicalis do not arise from the hypoglossal nerve. Instead, they "hitch a ride" with the hypoglossal nerve on the way to their final destination.

Veins of the Anterior Neck

Now that the musculature of the neck has been demonstrated and studied, attention may be turned to the arteries and veins of the neck.

After draining the face, the retromandibular vein travels inferiorly. Its anterior branch drains into a common trunk before ultimately draining into the internal jugular vein. Its posterior branch joins the posterior auricular vein forming the external jugular vein.

The external jugular vein lies directly over the sternocleidomastoid muscle before draining into the subclavian vein. Sometimes an anterior jugular vein joins the external jugular vein before the latter drains into the subclavian vein. Similarly, sometimes a communicating vein joins the external and anterior jugular veins over the surface of the sternocleidomastoid muscle.

The external jugular vein is very important since it can be readily viewed in the patient's neck when the patient is in a recumbent position. This vein is used to assist the clinician in assessing the patient's volume status and is particularly valuable in assessing patients in shock. Shock is an umbrella term used to describe any of a number of clinical conditions characterized by the inability of the body to deliver oxygenated blood to the tissues.

Arteries of the Anterior Neck

The majority of the head and neck are served by the common carotid artery.

The common carotid arteries arise from the aortic arch on the left side and the brachiocephalic trunk on the right side.

As the common carotid arteries ascend into the neck they become invested in fascia and become a part of the carotid sheaths. The common carotids bifurcate in the neck giving rise to the internal and external carotid arteries at the C4 vertebral level.

The internal carotid artery continues into the skull without giving off any branches in the neck.

The external carotid artery branches entirely in the neck eventually serving the face and neck, but nothing within the skull itself save the meninges. The meninges are served by the middle meningeal arteries which arise from the maxillary arteries which originate from the external carotid arteries.

At the point of bifurcation resides the carotid sinus and carotid body. The carotid sinus is a slight enlargement at the bifurcation point. It contains receptors which monitor blood pressure. Within the internal carotid artery near the bifurcation point resides the carotid body. The carotid body contains receptors which monitor oxygen and carbon dioxide levels in the blood. The carotid sinus and carotid body are innervated by cranial nerves nine and ten.

Lymphatics of the Anterior Neck

Capillaries are constantly allowing the filtration of fluids in and out of the vasculature through their walls. Normally, the amount of fluid filtered out of the capillaries is slightly larger than that which is allowed back into the capillaries. This fluid which remains in the interstitial spaces is returned to the circulation via lymphatic vessels which coalesce until they drain into the venous system.

Lymph nodes are tiny "stations" found along the lymphatic channels. They act to filter lymph and they also act to "test their environment" via resident white blood cells within. Ultimately, lymph nodes are important in the immune system's vigilant fight against internal and external pathology.

The jugulodigastric node is one of the major nodes through which most of the other nodes of the head drain. It serves as the beginning of the deep cervical lymph node chain which drains along the internal jugular vein. The jugulodigastric node can be found deep to the angle of the mandible.

Note also the submental lymph nodes inferior to the floor of the mouth and the submandibular lymph nodes inferior to the mandible. These nodes may be the first sites of metastatic spread in the patient with oral cancer. Indeed, the clinician may palpate enlarged nodes (with cancerous cells) before an oral lesion is even visible. This should underscore the importance of a complete and thorough head and neck examination at every appointment.

Sources Cited:

1-2. Brzezinski, et al. Laboratory and Study Guide for Head and Neck Anatomy: Dissection of the Head and Neck. Ann Arbor, MI. 2013

3-4. Gest, et al. Anatomy Tables (electronic MedCharts). Ann Arbor, MI. 2000

Laboratory Approach

☐1. Examine the superficial neck and dissect the skin (epidermis and dermis) exposing the platysma musculature within the hypodermis.

☐2. Examine the superficial layer of the deep cervical fascia (spanning the midline and investing the sternocleidomastoid muscles and the trapezius muscles) deep to the platysma.

☐3. Examine the sternocleidomastoid muscles deep to the platysma muscles.

☐4. Examine the infrahyoid muscles deep to the sternocleidomastoid muscles.

☐5. Examine and describe the anatomy of the cervical fascia.

☐6. Examine and describe the distribution and arrangement of the cervical plexus of nerves.

☐7. Examine and describe the distribution of the ansa cervicalis as it efferently serves the infrahyoid muscles.

☐8. Describe the various structures found within the anterior triangle and its subdivisions.

☐9. Examine and describe the anatomy of the thyroid gland.

☐10. Examine and describe the anatomy of the parathyroid glands.

☐11. Examine the carotid sheaths and their contents.

☐12. Examine and describe the deep cervical chain of lymph nodes running with the carotid sheaths.

☐13. Examine the osteology of the skull including the skull base, mandible, styloid processes and mastoid processes.

Cervical triangles
 Anterior
  Submental
  Submandibular
  Carotid
  Muscular
 Posterior
  Occipital
  Subclavian

Nerves
 Cervical plexus afferents (<u>cutaneous</u> branches)
  Lesser occipital, great auricular,
   transverse cervical (C2, 3)
  Supraclavicular (C3, 4)
 Cervical plexus efferents (<u>motor</u> branches)
  Ansa cervicalis (to strap mm.)
  Phrenic (C3, C4, C5)
 Facial (CN VII)
  Cervical branch
 Vagus (CN X)
 Spinal accessory (CN XI)
 Hypoglossal (CN XII)

Cervical veins
 Internal Jugular
  Retromandibular
   Posterior limb
   Anterior limb
 External jugular
 Communicating
 Anterior jugular
 Jugular venous arch
 Transverse cervical
 Suprascapular (deep to clavicle)
 Thyroid (superior, middle, and inferior)

Cervical Arteries
 Common carotid aa.
  Carotid sinus
  Carotid body
  External carotid
  Internal carotid
 Thyroid
  Superior thyroid
  Inferior thyroid

Muscles
  Platysma
  Infrahyoid ("strap")
    Sternohyoid
    Omohyoid (superior & inferior bellies)
    Sternothyroid
    Thyrohyoid
  Digastric (anterior and posterior bellies)
  Sternocleidomastoid (SCM)
  Trapezius

Deep cervical fascia
  Investing
  Infrahyoid (muscular)
  Visceral (pretracheal & retropharyngeal)
  Alar
  Prevertebral
  Carotid sheath

Central visceral compartment
  Thyroid Gland
    Isthmus
    Superior and inferior poles
    Pyramidal lobe
  Parathyroid Glands
  Trachea
  Esophagus

Cervical contents of carotid sheath
  Common carotid a.
  Internal jugular vein
  Vagus (CN X)
  Deep cervical chain of lymph nodes
  Ansa cervicalis (efferent cervical plexus fibers)

MASTOID PROCESS
MANDIBLE (Ramus, Angle, Base, Premasseteric Notch and Mental Symphysis)
HYOID BONE

Cartilaginous Structures

TRACHEAL RINGS
THYROID CARTILAGE (Lamina and Laryngeal Prominence)
CRICOID CARTILAGE

Posterior Neck

Introduction

This chapter will continue study of the neck with specific attention given to the posterior neck. The posterior neck contains the vertebral column, the spinal cord, the trapezius and levator scapulae muscles, and the deep musculature of the neck which surrounds and supports the vertebral column.

Besides being divided into anterior and posterior regions, recall that the neck can also be superficially divided into anterior and posterior triangles. The posterior triangle of the neck is bounded by the posterior border of the sternocleidomastoid muscle, the superior border of the clavicle, and the anterior border of the trapezius muscle. It can be further subdivided into the subclavian triangle and the occipital triangle. Similar to the anterior triangle and its subdivisions, the posterior triangle and its subdivisions allow scientists and clinicians to communicate effectively and to accurately describe the location of normal anatomy as well as pathology. By the end of the chapter you should be able to associate certain triangles with the structures that lie deep to them. Likely of primary importance is the fact that the subclavian (a.k.a. omohyoid) triangle has the subclavian vessels and the brachial plexus located deep to its surface.

The most important point to remember regarding the posterior neck is that in addition to containing the spinal column, it is also the location which contains the great nervous and vascular structures which serve the upper limbs. Sometimes scientists will consider this region the root of the neck. In all reality, the root of the neck is essentially the region inferior to the boundary between the anterior and posterior neck. It should be noted that any divisions in the neck are arbitrary and are intended only to aid in scientific communication and clinical care.

Posterior Neck Nerves

By way of review, the posterior portion of the head and neck are innervated by dorsal primary rami of the cervical nerves. The anterior neck is innervated by ventral primary rami of the cervical nerves.

Recall from the previous chapter that the cutaneous tissues of the anterior neck are innervated by nerve fibers from the cervical plexus of nerves. These fibers are ventral C2, C3, and C4 fibers. They arise deep from the spinal column (and their roots are thus posterior neck structures) and pass posterior to the posterior border of the sternocleidomastoid muscle at a small region called "Erb's Point" before coursing anteriorly to serve the anterior neck. These afferent nerves also serve the musculature of the anterior neck, including the sternocleidomastoid muscles, in order to give the central nervous system information regarding the location of the musculature in three-dimensional space.

The efferent fibers (ansa cervicalis fibers) arising from the cervical plexus are also ventral fibers. The ansa cervicalis is an anterior neck structure, but its roots arise deep from the spinal column. The roots are therefore posterior neck structures even though the more distal ansa cervicalis is an anterior neck structure. The ansa cervicalis efferently innervates the infrahyoid or strap muscles of the anterior neck.

Also passing posterior to the sternocleidomastoid muscle is the spinal accessory nerve (CN XI). The spinal accessory nerve, which is wholly efferent, originates in the posterior neck (just as the roots of the cervical plexus fibers do). It serves an anterior neck structure (sternocleidomastoid) as well as a posterior neck structure (trapezius). Its spinal roots enter the cranial cavity by passing up through the foramen magnum from the medulla oblongata and superior portion of the spinal cord and then exit the skull by passing through the jugular foramen with the internal jugular vein (as well as CN IX and CN X). (1, Nerves of the Head and Neck - Accessory)

The spinal accessory nerve can be found piercing the medial aspect of the sternocleidomastoid muscle and then emerging at the posterior border at or just below the upper and middle thirds of the sternocleidomastoid muscle before running obliquely down to the superior border of the trapezius muscle. The nerve is typically found in the superficial layer of deep cervical fascia (which invests both the sternocleidomastoids and the trapezius musculature). It should be noted that the spinal accessory nerve also passes over the surface of the levator scapulae muscle. The levator scapulae attaches to the transverse processes of the C1-C4 vertebrae and the scapula while serving to elevate the scapula (and is found posterior to the scalene muscles). (2, Muscles of the Head and Neck - Levator Scapulae)

The spinal accessory nerve efferently serves both the sternocleidomastoid muscle and the trapezius muscles. The trapezius has a diamond shape. It develops cervically before migrating to a more inferior position with its neurovascular supply. It elevates and depresses the scapula (depending on which part of the muscle contracts), rotates the scapula superiorly, and also retracts the scapula. (3, Muscles of the Upper Limb - Trapezius)

The nerve roots of the cervical plexus (C1-C4) and brachial plexus (C5-T1) are posterior neck structures arising from the spinal column. They are found in the laboratory setting by reflecting the sternocleidomastoid muscle and anterior scalene musculature forward and laterally. After reflection, the cervical spinal nerve roots may be found posterior to the carotid sheaths.

The Root of the Neck

The brachial plexus of nerves passes immediately posterior to the anterior scalene muscle and immediately anterior to the middle scalene muscle within the root of the neck.

The anterior scalene muscle is the key landmark in this region. Note that the phrenic nerve runs from superior to inferior across its anterior surface. Also note that the subclavian vein runs anterior to the anterior scalene muscle, while the subclavian artery and brachial plexus of nerves pass posterior to it. As the neurovasculature passes over the first rib they carve grooves into the bone.

The parasympathetic nervous system is represented in the root of the neck by the vagus nerve (CN X) within the carotid sheath. The vagus supplies parasympathetic innervation to most of the thorax and the proximal 2/3 of the gastrointestinal tract. The distal 1/3 of the gastrointestinal tract is parasympathetically supplied by the pelvic splanchnic nerves (S2-S4 parasympathetic outflow).

The sympathetic nervous system is represented in the root of the neck by the sympathetic trunk. Recall that the sympathetics arise from the spinal cord (T1-L2) and travel superiorly and inferiorly via the sympathetic trunk. The superior cervical ganglion is the highest point to which the sympathetic trunk travels. Sympathetic nerve fibers reach structures of the head and neck by traveling with the large arteries of the head and neck.

The top of the lungs may be located in the root of the neck. This superior-most portion of the lung's pleural lining is referred to as the cupola. Clinically its location at the root of the neck is important. Physicians sometimes need to gain access to the subclavian vessels at the root of the neck (to place a central line, etc.). The cupola of the lung may be iatrogenically damaged by needles or other objects if the clinician is not careful during his or her access procedures.

Sympathetic Trunk

In the last chapter on the anterior neck the carotid artery and its internal and external branches were examined. The internal carotid artery enters the skull base via the carotid canal (in the temporal bone). The internal jugular vein drains most of the blood from within the skull. It exits the skull through the jugular foramen. The vagus nerve also exits through this same foramen (as do the glossopharyngeal and spinal accessory nerves). The common carotid arteries, jugular veins, and vagus nerves are collectively wrapped in thick fascial investment known as the carotid sheaths. While technically a part of the anterior neck, the carotid sheaths are many times studied as posterior neck structures as well (which should confirm to the student the arbitrariness of the dividing lines between the anterior and posterior neck).

Note that the sympathetic trunk lies immediately medial to the carotid sheath, on or within the prevertebral fascia. The prevertebral fascia envelopes not only the neck muscles of the spinal column, but also the scalenes and the spinal nerve roots, including those of the brachial plexus.

The left and right cervical sympathetic trunks are a continuation of the thoracic sympathetic trunks and lie posterior and medial to the carotid sheath and anterior to the prevertebral muscles.

Consolidation of ganglia happens in the neck where there are only gray rami (as white rami are only found between T1 and L2 spinal levels). There are three cervical ganglia consolidations in the neck (the superior, middle, and inferior ganglia). There are only gray rami communicantes between the cervical sympathetic trunk and spinal nerves C1-C8 because the highest level for white rami is T1. All of the preganglionic fibers of the cervical sympathetic trunk originated at T1 or below (generally T1-T5) and all postganglionic fibers in the cervical sympathetic trunk originate from one of the three cervical ganglia.

The sympathetic innervation of the deep structures of the head and neck occurs via postganglionic sympathetic nerve fibers that follow branches of the external and internal carotid arteries.

The superior cervical ganglion sends postganglionic fibers via gray rami to C1-C4 spinal nerves. It can be found adjacent to the transverse process of the C2 vertebra. (4, Dissector Answers - Carotid Sheath, Pharynx, Larynx)

The middle cervical ganglion, which may or may not be present in all specimens, sends postganglionic fibers via gray rami to C5-6 spinal nerves. It is at the level of the C6 vertebra. (5,

Dissector Answers - Carotid Sheath, Pharynx, Larynx)

The cervicothoracic or stellate ganglion, the fusion of the inferior cervical and first thoracic ganglia, sends postganglionic fibers via gray rami to C6 - T1 spinal nerves. It can be found adjacent to the transverse process of C7. (6, Dissector Answers - Carotid Sheath, Pharynx, Larynx)

In general, sympathetic nerves cause contraction of smooth musculature leading to vasoconstriction and glandular secretion.

Specifically, the cervical sympathetic trunk controls:
- blood vessels of the head and neck
- blood vessels to midface and oral glands (including salivary glands)
- acceleration of heart rate and strength of cardiac contraction through superior, middle, and inferior cervical cardiac nerves
- innervation of hair muscles and sweat glands on the head and neck
- innervation of dilatator pupillae muscles of the eye and tarsal muscles of the eyelids (these allow iridial opening and palpebral fissure opening respectively) (7, Dissector Answers - Carotid Sheath, Pharynx, Larynx)

Horner's Syndrome is a constellation of signs and symptoms which arise when the sympathetic trunk is damaged.
- Since the iris is innervated by sympathetic fibers (via the short and long ciliary nerves in the orbit), any damage to these sympathetic fibers will result in *miosis* or pinpoint pupils (since the dilator pupillae musculature widens the iridial opening).
- Since the distal-most fibers of the levator palpebrae superioris (tarsal fibers) are sympathetically innervated, any damage to these sympathetic fibers will result in *ptosis* (drooping of the upper eyelid).
- The narrowed palpebral fissure will also give the appearance of *enophthalmos* (a deep-set eyeball).
- Damage to the sympathetic trunk will also result in an absence of sweating (*anhydrosis*) since the sweat glands are served by sympathetic fibers.

Subclavian Artery and Branches

The subclavian artery passes deep to the anterior scalene muscle and anterior to the middle scalene muscle within the interscalene triangle. Important branches of the subclavian artery include the thyrocervical trunk, the vertebral artery, the costocervical trunk, the internal thoracic artery, and the dorsal scapular artery.

The subclavian artery is typically subdivided into three parts according to the part's relationship to the anterior scalene muscle. The 1st PART has three branches: the vertebral artery, thyrocervical trunk (three branches: inferior thyroid, transverse cervical and suprascapular) and internal thoracic artery. The 2nd PART has one branch: the costocervical trunk. The 3rd PART has one branch: the dorsal scapular artery, which exists in 70% of the population. In the other 30% this artery arises from the transverse cervical artery.

The vertebral artery is examined elsewhere, but it is important to note here that it travels superiorly until it reaches the inside of the skull where it supplies the posterior portions of the cerebrum and surrounding structures.

The dorsal scapular artery arises from the 3rd PART of the subclavian artery and anastomoses with the suprascapular a. and the subscapular a. to form the scapular anastomoses. In nearly 1/3 of all cases the dorsal scapular a. arises from the transverse cervical a. The dorsal scapular nerve arises directly from the C5 spinal nerve root and innervates the levator scapulae m. and some other back muscles. (8, Arteries of the Upper Limb - Dorsal Scapular)

The suprascapular a. arises from the thyrocervical trunk and anastomoses with the circumflex scapular a. and the dorsal scapular a. to form the scapular anastomosis.

The subclavian artery becomes the axillary artery after it crosses over the first rib into the upper limb. An important artery, the lateral thoracic artery arises from the 2nd PART of the axillary artery and supplies the serratus anterior muscles of the thorax. The long thoracic nerve also supplies the serratus anterior muscles and arises from spinal nerves C5-C7 of the brachial plexus of nerves. Damage to its fibers leads to "winged scapula".

Subclavian steal syndrome is a term used to describe the retrograde flow of blood in the vertebral artery when the subclavian artery on the same side of the body (ipsilateral) is blocked and "steals" blood from the vertebral artery (causing retrograde flow). The subclavian artery is blocked before the vertebral artery arises allowing for the shunting of blood.

Clinically, if the subclavian artery is blocked proximal to the origination of the vertebral artery, use of the affected limb results in the shunting of blood from the Circle of Willis "backwards" through the vertebral artery to the subclavian artery where oxygen is most immediately needed. Such "stealing" of blood from the Circle of Willis to an upper limb may result in ischemia to the brain (and neurological sequela).

Thoracic Duct

The thoracic duct serves to drain all of the lymph of the body and limbs below the respiratory diaphragm. It also drains the left side of the chest, the left upper limb, and the left side of the head and neck above the diaphragm.

In traveling from an inferior to a superior position in the body, the thoracic duct passes through the diaphragm with the aorta. As it ascends in the abdominal and thoracic regions, it moves from the right side of the body over to the left side of the body. Its final destination is to drain into the venous circulation at the point where the left internal jugular vein and the left subclavian vein meet in the root of the neck. (9, Lymphatics of the Thorax - Thoracic Duct)

The lymph of the right side of the chest, the right upper limb, and the right side of the head and neck is drained via the right lymphatic duct. It typically drains into the venous circulation at the junction of the right internal jugular vein and the right subclavian vein in the root of the neck.

Sources Cited:

1-3, 8-9. Gest, et al. Anatomy Tables (electronic MedCharts). Ann Arbor, MI. 2000

4-7. Dissector Answers - Carotid Sheath, Pharynx, Larynx. 2000. http://www.med.umich.edu /lrc/coursepages/m1/anatomy2010/html/nervous_system/deepneck_ans.html.

Laboratory Approach

☐1. Examine the prevertebral fascia of the posterior neck as it invests the spinal column.

☐2. Examine the anterior, middle, and posterior scalene muscles. Describe the relationship between the scalenes and the neurovasculature of the root of the neck.

☐3. Examine the sternocleidomastoid and trapezius muscles. Be sure to also examine their neurovascular supply as well.

☐4. Examine and follow the course of the vagus (CN X) and spinal accessory (CN XI) nerves in the neck. Describe their functional significance.

☐5. Examine the sympathetic trunks and note their relationships to adjacent structures such as the spinal column and the carotid sheaths.

☐6. Examine and describe the subclavian blood vessels and their various parts and branches.

☐7. Examine the cervical plexus and note its deep origination from the spinal column.

☐8. Examine the brachial plexus and note its deep origination from the spinal column.

☐9. Examine the lymphatic drainage into the subclavian on the right (right lymphatic trunk) and the left (thoracic duct) sides.

☐10. Examine the bony vertebrae of the neck noting important specializations and processes.

Key Regional Structures

Nerves
    Brachial plexus (C5-T1)
    Cervical plexus afferents (<u>cutaneous</u> branches)
        Lesser occipital, great auricular,
            transverse cervical (C2, 3)
        Supraclavicular (C3, 4)
    Cervical plexus efferents (<u>motor</u> branches)
        Ansa cervicalis (to strap mm.)
        Phrenic (C3, C4, C5)
    Phrenic
    Suprascapular
    Facial (CN VII)
        Cervical branch
    Vagus (CN X)
    Spinal accessory (CN XI)
    Hypoglossal (CN XII)

Veins
    Internal jugular
    Subclavian
    Brachiocephalic
    Superior vena cava

Arteries
    Brachiocephalic
    Common carotid
    Subclavian
        <u>1st PART</u>
            Vertebral
            Thyrocervical trunk
                Inferior thyroid
                Ascending cervical
                Suprascapular
                Transverse cervical
                    (possible dorsal scapular coming off distally)
            Internal thoracic
        <u>2nd PART</u>
            Costocervical trunk
                Deep cervical
                Highest intercostal
        <u>3rd PART</u>
            Dorsal scapular (if not arising from transverse cervical)

Lymphatics
    Right lymphatic trunk
    Thoracic duct

Cervical sympathetic trunk
Superior, middle and inferior (cervicothoracic or stellate) ganglia
Ansa subclavia

Muscles
Anterior, middle and posterior scalene
Interscalene triangle

Miscellany
Prevertebral fascia
Cupola (superior-most extension of parietal pleura of lungs)

CERVICAL VERTEBRAE
SUPERIOR THORACIC APERTURE
1ST AND 2ND RIBS (Note: Pay special attention to bony attachment points for the scalene musculature as well as grooves marking the pathway of the subclavian vasculature.)

Superficial Face

Introduction

The subcutaneous muscles of the head and neck are considered facial muscles. This includes all the muscles of facial expression as well as the platysma (which was studied in a previous chapter on the neck). Embryologically, these muscles all arise from a common muscular sheet. As the musculature develops, individual groups are formed around the natural openings of the face (including the ears, eyes, nose and mouth). These muscles are all efferently innervated on their deep surfaces by branches of the facial nerve (CN VII). They originate deeply from bone or fascia and insert into the skin. When contracting together, these muscles allow the skin of the face to be moved and shaped into various expressions. They are also very important in other functions such as blinking (protection of the eye), opening and closing of the nasal openings, labial movements, speech, and the manipulation of food within the oral cavity. (1, p. 51) "Prior to the eruption of the dentition, facial muscles are integral to swallowing, and later, as the dentition erupts, the force of these muscles act in concert with the tongue to align the teeth within the dental arch." (2, p. 51)

All of the muscles of facial expression reside within the subcutaneous tissues and attach to the skin allowing movement of the skin upon contraction. Such actions of this musculature are vitally important in interpersonal communication. The interconnected system of facial musculature within the subcutaneous tissue is referred to as the SMAS (superficial muscular aponeurotic system) by surgeons.

While the cutaneous tissues of the face are afferently served by the trigeminal nerve branches (sensory innervation), the deeper muscles of facial expression are efferently served by branches of the facial nerve (motor innervation).

The muscles of facial expression provide certain surface anatomical landmarks. Of primary importance is the modiolus which lies immediately lateral to the corner (a.k.a. commissure or angle) of the mouth. It is here that multiple muscles of facial expression insert into the dermal layer of the overlying skin. These muscles are the zygomaticus major, risorius, platysma, depressor anguli oris, levator anguli oris, and buccinator muscles. The modiolus is commonly called the "dimple" when it is visible upon contraction of the involved musculature.

Facial Muscles

While the platysma was examined in the chapter relating to the anterior neck, it is actually one of the muscles of facial expression. The bulk of its fibers reside within the anterior neck, but its distal fibers pass superiorly over the base of the mandible and insert into the skin of the lower face. Recall that the platysma is efferently served by the cervical branch of the facial nerve (CN VII).

The muscles of facial expression are all efferently served by the facial nerve. They are afferently served (proprioceptively) by the trigeminal nerves which also pass through them in order to serve the skin as well.

When the platysma muscle is reflected, distal branches of the afferent cutaneous nerves from the cervical plexus are exposed. These nerves include the lesser occipital, great auricular, transverse cervical, and supraclavicular nerves. Recall that these nerves serve the tissues of the anterior neck and arise deep to the platysma along the posterior border of the sternocleidomastoid muscle from a small area called "Erb's Point".

The cervical branch of the facial nerve also travels deep to the platysma muscle entering at the muscle's posterior border near the angle of the mandible.

Another branch of the facial nerve travels deep to the platysma muscle. This branch is the marginal mandibular branch, and it lies immediately lateral to the facial artery and vein along the inferior border of the mandible. It serves to efferently innervate the musculature at the corner of the mouth.

The facial artery and vein are traveling from deep to superficial as they pass over the mandibular base in the premasseteric notch. Notice specifically that the artery lies anterior to the vein.

The parotid gland is the largest salivary gland in the body, and it is found overlying the ramus and angle of the mandible. It extends deeply posterior to the ramus of the mandible, and it may also be found inferior to the angle of the mandible immediately anterior to the sternocleidomastoid muscle. It is noted here because the branches of the facial nerve which serve the muscles of facial expression pass through the substance of the parotid gland as they travel from the stylomastoid foramen (in the skull base) to their target muscles. The parotid ducts, which carry saliva from the glands to intraoral openings, can be seen traveling lateral to the masseter muscles before penetrating through the buccinator muscles. As an aside, the masseter muscles are muscles of mastication and allow for chewing of food and elevation of the mandible. They are efferently innervated by motor branches of V3 and will be studied later in this book.

Notice that the parotid duct pierces through the buccinator muscle (a muscle of facial expression) before arriving in the oral cavity. While the buccinator muscle is a muscle of facial expression, it is also vitally important in mastication as it assists the tongue in keeping food upon the occlusal table (between the teeth). The buccinator attaches at the modiolus and passes posteriorly before attaching to fibers of the superior pharyngeal constrictor muscles at the pterygomandibular raphae. Together the buccinator and superior constrictor muscles create a "horseshoe" shaped column of muscles which define the boundaries of the oral cavity and oral pharynx.

The depressor labii inferioris and platysma act at the inferior border of the lips and retract the lips downward. This can be clinically assessed by asking the patient to "curl" their lower lip inferiorly. The cervical and marginal mandibular branches innervate these muscles.

The depressor anguli oris acts at the corners of the mouth and allows the patient to "frown". The marginal mandibular and buccal branches innervate these muscles.

The orbicularis oris completely encircles the oral opening and allows the patient to "purse" his or her lips. The buccal branches innervate this set of muscles.

The mentalis acts to retract the lower lip downward and is innervated by the marginal mandibular branch of the facial nerve.

The levator labii superioris acts to elevate the upper lip and is innervated by the buccal branches of the facial nerve.

The buccinator pulls the corner of the mouth laterally and is innervated by the buccal branches of the facial nerve. This can be assessed by asking the patient to "puff" out his or her cheeks against external resistance.

The orbicularis oculi acts to close the eyelids and is innervated by the temporal and zygomatic branches of the facial nerve.

The frontalis acts to raise the eyebrows and is innervated by the temporal branch of the facial nerve.

The function of the facial nerve and the musculature it efferently innervates can be assessed easily by asking the patient to perform specific actions.

Facial Nerve

The facial nerve arises from the pons and begins its exit from the skull through the internal acoustic meatus. It carries autonomic and somatic nerve fibers at its start.

The autonomic fibers of the facial nerve split off from the remaining somatic fibers within the temporal bone of the skull. They will be studied at a later time.

The remaining somatic fibers leave the skull via the stylomastoid foramen and are entirely efferent. The stylomastoid foramen lies between the styloid process and mastoid process on the external skull base. At this point these efferent somatic fibers are destined to serve the muscles of facial expression and pass out of the skull deep to the parotid gland. They then pass through the parotid gland before reaching their target muscles. Clinically this is important since parotidectomy (removal of the parotid gland) is tedious as each and every branch of the facial nerve must be isolated and spared.

The most superior branch of the facial nerve is the temporal branch. It travels to the lateral aspect of the skull over the temporal bone.

Slightly anterior and inferior to the temporal branch is the zygomatic branch of the facial nerve. It travels to the musculature at the lateral angle of the orbit (where the eye resides).

Inferior to the zygomatic branch is the buccal branch of the facial nerve which overlies the buccinator muscle.

Inferior to the buccal branch of the facial nerve is the marginal mandibular branch. It is found at the base of the mandible immediately lateral to the facial vessels. This is clinically important because one can reflect the marginal mandibular branch laterally if one also reflects the facial vessels laterally. This intraoperative "pearl" is very useful if one needs to access the mandible surgically.

The most inferiorly placed branch of the facial nerve is the cervical branch, and it is found below the mandible as it travels anteriorly to efferently innervate the platysma muscle.

Bell's Palsy (named for its discoverer, Dr. Charles Bell) is a relatively common condition which affects the efferent fibers of the facial nerve. This palsy results in the ipsilateral paralysis of one side of the face (both upper and lower face). Bell's can be differentiated from a central deficit (such as a stroke) by demonstrating the patient's inability to raise the eyebrow on the affected side since central deficits affect only the lower face (due to complex crossing patterns of the fibers before the stylomastoid foramen). Bell's Palsies are typically of an unknown etiology (with inflammation of CN VII at its exit point being the most likely underlying cause). Symptoms resolve on their own without specific treatment within a few weeks while complete resolution is usually seen within 6 months. The patient's primary complaints include the inability to close the eye on the affected side and the inability to keep the corner of the mouth closed ("dry eye" and "drooling" on the affected side). However, all ipsilateral facial muscles are affected.

Trigeminal Nerve

The various dermatomes (innervated by afferent cutaneous or sensory nerves) of the face and neck have already been touched upon in other places. The cervical plexus afferently serves the tissues of the neck while the trigeminal nerve (CN V) afferently serves the tissues of the face.

By way of review, note specifically that the upper eyelid, nasal bridge, and forehead are served by the ophthalmic nerve (V1). The lower eyelid and upper lip are served by the maxillary nerve (V2). The lower lip and base of the mandible are served by the mandibular nerve (V3).

Note also that V1, V2, and V3 can be further divided into specific named nerve branches.

The primary V1 branches are the supraorbital, supratrochlear, infratrochlear, and lacrimal nerves which serve the area above the orbit and upper eyelids. The external nasal nerve serves the bridge of the nose.

The primary V2 branches are the zygomaticotemporal and zygomaticofacial nerves which serve the lateral upper face. The infraorbital nerve serves the midface region between the lower eyelid and the upper lip.

The primary V3 branches are the buccal nerve (NOT the buccal branch of the facial nerve) and the mental nerve which serve the lateral aspect of the mandible and lower lip (respectively). The auriculotemporal nerve is also a branch of V3 and is found on the lateral aspect of the upper mandible (as well as the temporal region of the skull).

The branches of the trigeminal nerve DO NOT efferently innervate any muscles of facial expression. They are afferent and sensory (NOT efferent and motor) nerves.

Note that the efferent facial nerve branches are found in close proximity to the afferent trigeminal nerve branches. In fact, it is not uncommon for trigeminal nerve fibers to "hitch a ride" on the motor branches of the facial nerve since they are traveling in the same regions.

Recall that the trigeminal and facial nerves both arise from the pons portion of the brainstem.

Vascular Supply of the Face

Recall that the facial vessels (artery and vein) are found in the premasseteric notch anterior to the parotid gland and the masseter muscle.

The facial artery originates in the upper neck as it arises from the external carotid artery. It branches from the external carotid artery superior to the superior thyroid branch and courses superoanteriorly along the external floor of the mouth until it passes through the capsule of the submandibular gland. Once at the premasseteric notch it travels superiorly (anterior to the facial vein) over the lateral aspect of the face. Branches come off from it to serve the upper and lower lips as well as the medial aspect of the orbit.

The facial vein mirrors the course of the facial artery, but drains its contents into the internal jugular vein. Its course is unique in that it is posterior to the artery, and does NOT travel through the submandibular capsule. Instead, it remains lateral to the capsule and gland.

The remaining arterial supply to the face (all of which arises from the external carotid artery) will be studied later in this book when the face is dissected more deeply. Most of the deeper facial structures are served by branches of the maxillary artery which is one of two terminal branches of the external carotid artery. The other terminal branch of the external carotid artery is the superficial temporal artery. It can be found immediately anterior to the ear and travels superiorly along the lateral aspect of the skull with the auriculotemporal nerve (branch of V3).

As a general rule, there are lymphatic vessels and lymph nodes wherever there are veins. It follows, therefore, that there are superficial and deep sets of lymphatic nodes and vessels just as there are superficial and deep sets of veins. Nodes of the face ultimately drain into superficial and deep cervical lymph nodes.

Sources Cited:

1-2. Brzezinski, et al. Laboratory and Study Guide for Head and Neck Anatomy: Dissection of the Head and Neck. Ann Arbor, MI. 2013

Laboratory Approach

☐1. Examine the scalp and review its layers.

☐2. Examine the superficial muscles of facial expression and identify their neurovasculature and attachment points.

☐3. Examine the bony anatomy of the face and mandible. Identify important structures on the mandible.

☐4. Examine the facial nerve and outline its various branches which serve to efferently innervate the musculature of the face.

☐5. Examine the trigeminal nerve and outline its various branches which serve to afferently innervate the soft tissues of the face.

☐6. Examine the buccal fat pad and describe its mechanistic and functional roles.

☐7. Examine the buccinator muscle and understand its neurovasculature and functional role in facial expression and mastication.

☐8. Describe the vasculature of the face with particular attention paid to the facial artery and vein (which can be found within the premasseteric notch).

☐9. Examine the osteology of the face with particular attention paid to the mandible.

Muscles of facial expression:
    Scalp muscles
      occipitofrontalis (epicranius)
        frontalis
        occipitalis
        galea aponeurotica

    External ear muscles
      ant., sup. & post. auricular

    Eyelid muscles
      orbicularis oculi
        orbital portion
        palpebral portion
      corrugator supercilii

    Perioral muscles
      muscles attaching to modiolus
        orbicularis oris
        buccinator
        zygomaticus major
        risorius
        platysma
        depressor anguli oris
        levator anguli oris

      muscles inserting between modiolus & midline
        zygomaticus minor
        levator labii superioris
        levator labii superioris alaeque nasi
        depressor labii inferioris
        mentalis

    Nasal muscles
      nasalis
      compressor naris
      dilator naris

Vessels
    Superficial temporal a. & v.
    Facial a. & v.
      superior labial branch
      inferior labial branch
      lateral nasal branch
    Angular a. & v.
    Deep facial v.

Nerves
    Auriculotemporal n.
    Greater & lesser occipital nn.
    Great auricular n.
    Trigeminal n. (CN V)
        Ophthalmic division (V1)
       frontal n. (present in orbit)
        supraorbital n.
          medial branch
          lateral branch
        supratrochlear n.
      nasociliary n. (present in orbit)
        infratrochlear n.
        external nasal n.
      lacrimal n.
      Maxillary division (V2)
      infraorbital n.
      zygomaticotemporal n.
      zygomaticofacial n.
      Mandibular division (V3)
      auriculotemporal n.
      mental n.
      buccal n. (long buccal n.)

Miscellaneous
    Ala of nose
    Nasal columella
    Philtrum
    Nasolabial fold
    Mentolabial fold
    Buccal fat pad
    Pterygomandibular raphe

ALVEOLAR PROCESSES of MAXILLA & MANDIBLE
BUCCAL SHELF of MANDIBLE
APEX of RETROMOLAR TRIGONE
HAMULUS of MEDIAL PTERYGOID PLATE
MENTAL FORAMEN
INFRAORBITAL FORAMEN
SUPRAORBITAL FORAMEN (or NOTCH)
ZYGOMATICOFACIAL FORAMEN
ZYGOMATICOTEMPORAL FORAMEN
GROOVE for EXTERNAL NASAL NERVE (on the deep surface of nasal bone)

Review the bones of the skull. Specifically study the facial bones and mandible this session. The mandible has special anatomic features which are particularly important to the clinician specializing in the oral cavity.

MANDIBLE
>   Body
>   Ramus
>   Angle
>   Coronoid process
>   Condyle
>   Neck
>   Temporal crest
>   Oblique line
>   Mental foramen
>   Mandibular canal
>   Alveolar arch
>   Mylohyoid groove
>   Mylohyoid line
>   Pterygoid fovea
>   Submandibular fossa
>   Sublingual fossa
>   Digastric fossa
>   Mental spines
>   Lingula
>   Mandibular foramen
>   Mental protuberance
>   Mandibular notch

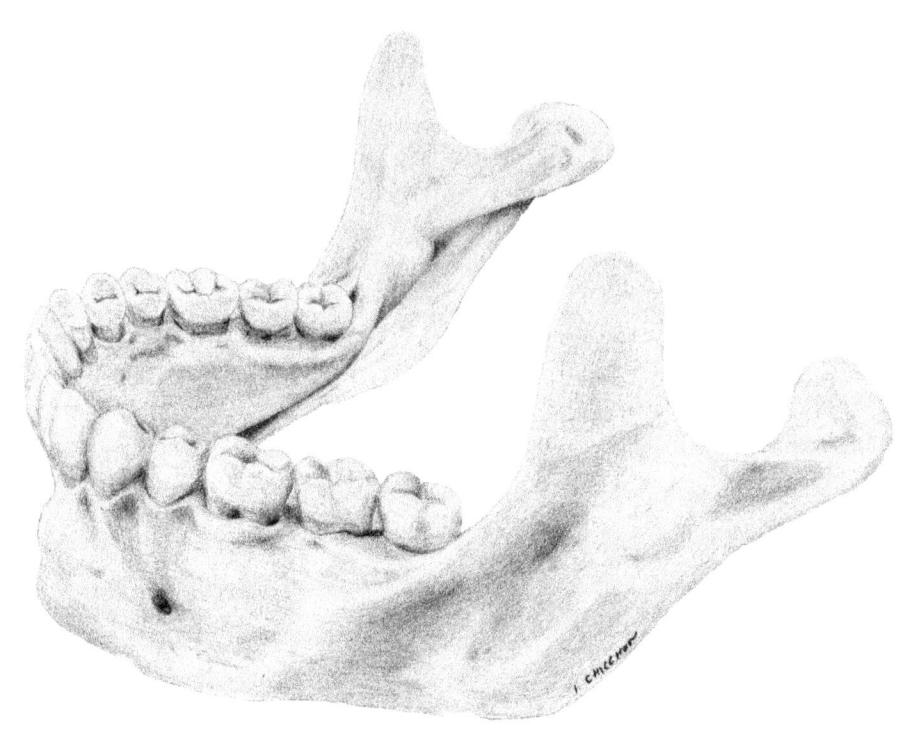

Lateral Face and the Parotid Gland

Introduction

The superficial face and muscles of facial expression were examined in the previous chapter. This chapter will review many of the same structures, but will focus more attention on the parotid gland.

Lateral Face

The parotid gland can be found overlying the ramus and angle of the mandible. The gland typically also extends posterior, deep, and inferior to the mandible. Small superficial veins pass through the substance of the gland, as do the motor branches of the facial nerve. The parotid duct can be seen passing anteriorly from the parotid gland over the masseter muscle before diving through the buccinator to empty into the oral cavity lateral to the maxillary 2nd molar.

The facial artery and vein which were studied in the previous chapter can also be seen in the premasseteric notch.

The motor fibers of the facial nerve exit the temporal bone via the stylomastoid foramen. Note that the autonomic fibers of the facial nerve exit temporal bone earlier and will be studied later in this book.

Besides sending branches to the muscles of facial expression already studied, the facial nerve sends other branches to additional structures. One such branch (the posterior auricular nerve) travels posterior to the ear to efferently innervate the occipitalis and posterior auricularis muscles. Another such branch efferently innervates the posterior bellies of the digastric muscles and the stylohyoid muscles. The digastric and stylohyoid muscles will be studied in more detail later in the book.

The most superior branch of the facial nerve is the temporal branch. It travels to the lateral aspect of the skull over the temporal bone innervating the anterior auricularis muscle and the frontalis muscle bellies.

Slightly anterior and inferior to the temporal branch is the zygomatic branch of the facial nerve. It travels to the musculature at the lateral angle of the orbit (where the eye resides) innervating the orbicularis oculi.

Inferior to the zygomatic branch is the buccal branch of the facial nerve which overlies the buccinator muscle innervating muscles of facial expression in the midface region.

Inferior to the buccal branch of the facial nerve is the marginal mandibular branch. It is found at the base of the mandible immediately lateral to the facial vessels. Recall that this is clinically important because one can reflect the marginal mandibular branch laterally if one also reflects the facial vessels laterally. This nerve efferently innervates musculature at the corner of the mouth and the lower lip.

The most inferiorly placed branch of the facial nerve is the cervical branch, and it is found below the mandible as it travels anteriorly to efferently innervate the platysma muscle.

It is common for the superior-most portions of the facial nerve to be "lumped together". The temporal, zygomatic, and superior buccal branches are typically grouped and referred to as the *temporofacial division* of the facial nerve. These nerves collectively innervate the muscles of facial expression on the upper part of the face (frontalis muscle, anterior and superior auricularis muscles, and the orbicularis oculi muscles). The inferior buccal, marginal mandibular, and cervical branches are typically grouped and referred to as the *cervicofacial division* of the facial nerve. These nerves collectively innervate the muscles of facial expression on the lower part of the face (including the platysma muscle).

The cervicofacial division usually forms a loop by communicating with the temporofacial division of the facial nerve.

Skull Base

Of particular importance in this region is the location of the styloid and mastoid processes on the skull base. Recall that the stylomastoid foramen resides between these two bony landmarks and is the exit point of the motor fibers of the facial nerve (CN VII). Both processes and the stylomastoid foramen are found within temporal bone of the skull.

Other foramina and openings in the same region should be studied at this point and will be discussed at other points in this book. For example, the petrotympanic fissure is found anterior to the stylomastoid foramen (within the mandibular fossa) and the tympanic canaliculus is found anteromedially to the stylomastoid foramen. These two openings allow for the passage of preganglionic parasympathetic fibers (from CN VII and IX respectively).

You should note that the mandibular fossa (which contains the condylar head of the mandible) is directly anterior and lateral to the stylomastoid foramen.

Parotid Gland

"The parotid gland resides within a wedge-shaped, fascial fossa which lies between the ramus of the mandible and the anterior border of the sternocleidomastoid muscle." (1, p. 67) The gland passes anteriorly over the lateral border of the masseter muscle, and both structures (gland and muscle) are covered by the parotidomasseteric fascia which is an extension of the investing layer of the deep cervical fascia. (2, p. 67)

The parotidomasseteric fascia can be found attached to the zygomatic arch and maxilla superiorly, and the mandible inferiorly. (3, p. 67)

Another specialization of the investing layer of the deep cervical fascia is the angular tract. This portion of deep cervical fascia is found passing between the angle of the mandible and the anterior border of the sternocleidomastoid muscle. This tract of fascia separates the parotid gland from the more inferiorly placed submandibular gland. (4, p. 67)

Continuous with, and ascending superior to the angular tract is a deep portion of the deep cervical fascia which attaches to the temporal bone of the skull base.

- The portion of this deep cervical fascia which spans between the anterior border of the sternocleidomastoid muscle and the styloid process (temporal bone) forms the *posterior deep wall* of the parotid gland fossa. It is important to note that the stylohyoid muscle and posterior belly of the digastric muscle are traveling within (and are enclosed by) this sheet of deep cervical fascia. (5, p. 67)
- Another portion of this deep cervical fascia spans between the styloid process and the posterior border of the ramus of the mandible forming the *anterior deep wall* of the parotid gland fossa (a.k.a. the stylomandibular ligament and membrane). (6, p. 67)

In general, the parotid gland lies lateral to the ramus of the mandible and the masseter muscle. It also lies deep to the posterior border of the mandible in the parotid fossa and anterior to the anterior border of the sternocleidomastoid muscle.

The important structures which pass through the parotid gland are the external carotid artery, the retromandibular vein and the facial nerves (which is superficial to the vasculature within the gland).

The external carotid artery passes through the parotid gland and gives off the superficial temporal artery (the proximal portion of which is also located in the parotid gland).

The superficial temporal vein drains into the retromandibular vein before its split into the anterior and posterior retromandibular veins.

The temporal, zygomatic, buccal, marginal mandibular, and cervical branches of the facial nerve can also be seen passing through the gland on their way to supply the muscles of facial expression. The facial nerve branches pass through the parotid in one plane, thus dividing the gland into a superficial and a deep portion.

Parotid Gland Pathology

On the medial (deep and internal) side of the ramus of the mandible, and immediately anterior to the deep portion of the parotid gland, one finds branches of V3 exiting the skull from the foramen ovale (within the infratemporal fossa) and entering the oral cavity. These nerves will be studied in great detail later in the book, but it is important to recognize that these are the primary afferent nerves which innervate the mandibular teeth and the lower oral cavity.

This region is very important clinically since the dentist anesthetizes the branches of V3 (and the inferior alveolar nerve in particular) when he or she performs work on the mandibular teeth. It is not uncommon for the dentist to accidentally direct the needle too far posteriorly and inject local anesthetic into the parotid fossa posterior to the ramus of the mandible. If this occurs, the patient will suffer a transient paralysis of the facial nerve since the facial nerve passes through the substance of the parotid gland.

Another relatively common problem is inflammation of the parotid gland secondary to infection with a virus (such as the mumps virus). The parotid glands may also be bilaterally enlarged in patients taking anti-histamine medications.

Mumps parotitis can be very serious, but the vaccine was licensed in the 1960s and there are now many fewer cases in the United States. It is still, however, common in other parts of the world. Symptoms include swollen painful parotid glands (on one or both sides of the face), pain with mastication (chewing), fever, and generalized weakness. The virus is spread person to person via contaminated saliva. Serious complications include orchitis (testicular swelling and inflammation, which may lead to infertility in affected teenagers), pancreatitis, encephalitis, meningitis, ovarian inflammation, hearing loss, and miscarriage. (7, Pasternack, 2013)

Review of the Nerves of the Face

The facial nerve contains autonomic fibers at its inception point. These fibers are parasympathetic and travel to the pterygopalatine (sphenopalatine) ganglion and the submandibular ganglion. They split off from the rest of the facial nerve fibers within the temporal bone and will ultimately innervate various glands of the orbit, midface, and oral cavity.

Another small branch of the facial nerve (within the chorda tympani) supplies taste sensation to the anterior two-thirds of the tongue.

To summarize, the facial nerve arises from the pons and contains motor, autonomic, and special taste fibers. The motor fibers were discussed in a previous chapter, and the autonomic and taste fibers will be studied in more detail later in the book.

The trigeminal nerve serves the entire face afferently and its three major branches (V1, V2, and V3) split the face up into distinct dermatomes. These dermatomes are clinically important. Their importance can be illustrated with a brief examination of Herpes Zoster. Herpes Zoster (a.k.a. "Shingles") is the reactivation of the varicella-zoster virus (a.k.a. "Chickenpox").

Following recovery from the Chickenpox the varicella-zoster virus can enter the nervous system and remain dormant for many years. After some time it may reactivate and travel along the nerves to the skin to produce Shingles.

The reactivation affects only a specific dermatome (one particular set of nerve fibers) and may appear anywhere on the body (unilaterally). The head and neck clinician may see the V1, V2, or V3 dermatome affected.

Signs and symptoms of Herpes Zoster infection include pruritis, pain, burning, numbness, and tingling over the affected area. A red rash forms a few days following the onset of the pain, and it is followed by blisters which ooze before eventually crusting over.

Autonomic Innervation of the Parotid Gland

The glossopharyngeal nerve (CN IX) arises from the medulla and leaves the skull via the jugular foramen. Its primary role is to afferently serve the posterior portion of the pharynx.

Immediately following its exit from the skull, a small set of fibers (the tympanic nerve) split off from the glossopharyngeal nerve. These fibers travel superiorly right back up into the skull through the tympanic canaliculus (found directly between the jugular foramen and the carotid canal).

These preganglionic parasympathetic fibers travel through the middle ear space before leaving the temporal bone of the skull by means of the lesser petrosal nerve. The lesser petrosal nerve then travels over the internal skull base before exiting through the foramen ovale adjacent to the mandibular branch of the trigeminal nerve.

The preganglionic fibers then synapse in the otic ganglion which is found immediately medial to the trunk of mandibular branch of the trigeminal nerve after it has exited the skull base.

Postganglionic fibers exit the otic ganglion and hitch a ride on the auriculotemporal nerve before finally jumping off in the substance of the parotid gland to innervate it.

Carotid Triangle Review

Recall that the carotid triangle is a smaller triangle found within the anterior triangle of the neck. It is bounded posteriorly by the anterior border of the sternocleidomastoid muscle, anteriorly by the superior belly of the omohyoid muscle, and superiorly by the posterior belly of the digastric muscle.

There are various nerves within the carotid triangle. Portions of the vagus nerve, spinal accessory nerve, and hypoglossal nerves can all be found within the carotid triangle. The superior ramus of the ansa cervicalis is also found within the carotid triangle. Recall that the ansa cervicalis and the nerve to the thyrohyoid appear to arise from the hypoglossal nerve. They do not. They merely hitch a ride with the hypoglossal nerve but are originally derived from the cervical plexus of nerves.

As previously mentioned, the internal jugular vein is also within the carotid triangle.

It is within the carotid triangle that the lingual, facial, and superior thyroid veins drain into the internal jugular vein. Recall that the facial vein is found within the premasseteric notch (posterior to the facial artery).

The primary significance of the carotid triangle may be that the carotid artery splits within this triangle. The carotid sheath is also found here.

It is also within the carotid triangle that the lingual, facial, and superior thyroid artery branch off from the external carotid artery.

There are no branches of the internal carotid artery within the carotid triangle. In fact, there are no branches of the internal carotid artery anywhere within the neck. The first branches off from the internal carotid artery occur within the skull.

The first branch off from the anterior aspect of the external carotid artery is the superior thyroid artery which descends to serve the superior poles of the thyroid gland.

Next, the ascending pharyngeal artery branches off from the posterior aspect of the external carotid artery to supply the pharyngeal wall.

The occipital artery also branches off from the posterior aspect of the external carotid artery, but does so more superiorly. This artery passes along the inferior border of the posterior belly of the digastric muscle before passing medial to the origin of the muscle.

The posterior auricular artery originates in the lower portion of the parotid fossa and runs along the superior border of the posterior belly of the digastric muscle. It is important in that a small branch (the stylomastoid branch) supplies the facial nerve within the temporal bone.

Superior to the anterior branch point of the superior thyroid artery one finds the lingual and facial arteries branching from the external carotid artery. It should be noted that sometimes these two arteries (lingual and facial) arise from a common trunk on the anterior surface of the external carotid artery. The lingual artery can always be found passing deep to the hyoglossus muscle at the superior border of the greater horn of the hyoid bone.

Before the external carotid artery terminates into the maxillary and superficial temporal arteries, a small posterior auricular branch is given off from its posterior surface to ultimately serve the area posterior to the ear.

Sources Cited:

1-6. Brzezinski, et al. Laboratory and Study Guide for Head and Neck Anatomy: Dissection of the Head and Neck. Ann Arbor, MI. 2013

7. Pasternack M. 2013. What Everyone Should Know About Mumps. MassGeneral Hospital For Children News. [accessed 2014 July 20]. http://www.massgeneral.org/children/about/newsarticle.aspx?id=4178]

Laboratory Approach

☐1. Examine the parotid gland and its fossa bed.

☐2. Examine the neurovasculature which passes through the parotid gland.

☐3. Examine the course of the facial nerve as it arises from the stylomastoid foramen deep to the parotid fossa and then distributes distally to the muscles of facial expression.

☐4. Review the boundaries of the carotid triangle.

☐5. Identify the contents of the carotid triangle.

☐6. Identify and examine the branches of the external carotid artery and study their distribution and the structures they serve.

☐7. Review the osteology of the face.

Key Regional Structures

Parotid Gland
    Fascial boundaries
        parotidomasseteric fascia
        angular tract of fascia
                (interglandular septum)
        anterior deep wall
            (stylomandibular lig. & membrane)
        posterior deep wall
    Body of gland
    Accessory parotid gland
    Parotid duct and papilla

Nerves
        Facial nerve (CN VII) (in the face and neck)
        Posterior auricular br.
        Nerve to posterior digastric muscle
        Nerve to stylohyoid muscle
        Parotid plexus of nn.
            temporofacial division
              temporal bb.
              zygomatic bb.
              buccal bb.
            cervicofacial division (inconstant)
              buccal bb.
              mandibular (and marginal) bb.
              cervical b.

        Other Regional Cranial nerves
        Trigeminal (V3)
            mylohyoid n.
            nerve to anterior digastric muscles
            auriculotemporal n.
        Vagus (CN X)
            superior laryngeal branch
        Accessory (CN XI)
        Hypoglossal (CN XII)

    Sensory nerves
    Cervical plexus nn.

Autonomic nervous system
    Sympathetic
        superior cervical ganglion
    Parasympathetic
        glossopharyngeal n. (IX)
            tympanic branch
        tympanic plexus
        lesser petrosal n.
            otic ganglion

Cervical triangles (Review)
    Carotid
    Submandibular
    Submental

Arteries
    External Carotid
      Superior thyroid a.
        superior laryngeal a.
        infrahyoid a.
      Ascending pharyngeal a.
      Lingual a.
        suprahyoid a.
      Facial a.
        ascending palatine a.
        submental a.
      Occipital a.
      Posterior auricular a.
        stylomastoid a.

Veins
    Internal jugular vein
      Superior thyroid v.
      Lingual v.
       (& vena comitans hypoglossi)
      Facial (or common facial) v.
      Pharyngeal vv.
    Retromandibular vein (anterior and posterior divisions)
      Superficial temporal v.
      Maxillary v.
    Facial v. (and "common facial v.")

Muscles
    Anterior & posterior bellies of digastric m.
    Stylohyoid
    Mylohyoid (& raphe)
    Hyoglossus

Miscellaneous
    Submandibular gland (superficial lobe)
    Submandibular & submental lymph nodes

Osteology

In this and subsequent chapters relevant bones of the skull and face will be examined in detail. The mandible was covered in the previous chapter. Eventually, all of the bones of the face will be studied in detail.

FRONTAL BONE
Zygomatic process
Temporal line
Orbital plates
Frontal sinus
Sulcus for superior sagittal sinus
Frontal eminence
Superciliary arches
Supraorbital margin
Supraorbital foramen
Fossa for lacrimal gland
Trochlear fovea
Nasal process
Anterior and posterior ethmoidal foramina

PARIETAL BONE
Coronal suture
Parietal eminence
Parietal foramen
Lambdoidal suture
Granular foveae
Sagittal sulcus
Sulci for meningeal aa.
Superior temporal line
Inferior temporal line

OCCIPITAL BONE
Lambdoidal suture
Superior nuchal line
Basilar portion
Jugular notch
Occipital condyles
Internal occipital protuberance
External occipital protuberance
Pharyngeal tubercle
Hypoglossal canal
Occipital squama
Groove for superior sagittal sinus
Foramen magnum
Condyloid canal

ZYGOMATIC BONE
    Malar surface
    Orbital surface
    Maxillary process
    Temporal surface
    Temporal process
    Frontal process
    Zygomaticofacial foramen
    Zygomaticotemporal foramen
    Zygomaticoorbital foramen (or foramina)

PALATINE BONE
    Horizontal plate
    Pyramidal process
    Vertical plate
    Palatine crest
    Orbital process (in combination with maxilla)
    Greater & lesser palatine canals (inferior termination of the pterygopalatine canal)
    Posterior nasal spine
    Pterygopalatine groove
    Sphenopalatine notch
    Greater palatine foramen
    Lesser palatine foramen

HYOID BONE
    Body
    Greater horn
    Lesser horn

Tongue and the Paralingual Space

<u>Introduction</u>

Topics covered in this chapter include the floor of the mouth, the submandibular and sublingual triangles, the paralingual space, and the tongue.

<u>Extraoral Floor of the Mouth</u>

Deep to the platysma muscles (but superficial to the mylohyoid musculature) at the base of the mandible lie the digastric muscles. The digastric muscles serve to elevate the hyoid bone and depress the mandible (in concert with the lateral pterygoid muscles and other muscles of the floor of the mouth). The digastric muscles have two bellies: an anterior and a posterior belly. The anterior belly of the digastric muscle is efferently innervated by motor fibers of the mandibular division of the trigeminal nerve (V3) by way of the mylohyoid nerve. The posterior belly is efferently innervated by motor fibers of the facial nerve (CN VII).

It is important to note that the digastric muscles were formed (embryologically) from mesenchyme originating from the first two pharyngeal arches. This dual origin (two distinct pharyngeal arches) is the reason for the dual innervation (with the anterior belly innervated by CN V3 and the posterior belly innervated by CN VII).

The stylohyoid muscles lie lateral to the facial arteries and hypoglossal nerves. The stylohyoid muscle elevates and retracts the hyoid bone. It splits around the intermediate tendon of the digastric muscle before attaching to the body of the hyoid bone. Both the stylohyoid muscle and the posterior belly of the digastric muscle are efferently innervated by motor fibers of the facial nerve.

The digastric muscles and the stylohyoid muscles are extraoral muscles which assist in the creation of the floor of the mouth. The digastric bellies are also important as they mark the boundaries of the submandibular and sublingual triangles which will be studied in more detail during this chapter.

Both the submandibular and sublingual triangles are inferior to the floor of the mouth and are smaller triangles which lie within the larger anterior triangle. They are superficial triangles.

The submandibular triangle is found immediately inferior to the mylohyoid muscle, and the superficial portion of the submandibular gland is found within the triangle.

The submandibular gland has both a deep and superficial portion. The deep portion is in the paralingual space superior to the mylohyoid muscle at its posterolateral border. The superficial portion is in the submandibular triangle inferior to the mylohyoid muscle.

<u>Submandibular and Sublingual Triangles</u>

Time should now be taken to review the boundaries of the anterior triangle as well as all of its subdivisions (the smaller triangles it contains). This content was covered in the chapter on the anterior neck.

The most important structures found within the submandibular triangle are the submandibular gland and the facial artery and vein. The triangle, however, also contains the mylohyoid nerve (which efferently innervates the mylohyoid muscle of the floor of the mouth and ultimately arises from the inferior alveolar nerve, a branch of the mandibular division of the trigeminal nerve) and the hypoglossal nerve.

The submandibular glands are classified as "major salivary glands" (along with the parotid glands and the sublingual glands). They are located below the mylohyoid muscle in the submandibular triangle and are innervated by parasympathetic fibers passing through the submandibular ganglion in the paralingual space. These autonomic fibers originate from the facial nerve and travel to the submandibular ganglion via the chorda tympani nerve.

The submandibular glands and sublingual glands are "mixed" salivary glands meaning that they produce a product that is both serous and mucinous. The submandibular gland, however, is primarily serous. The sublingual glands are primarily mucinous. Both are mixed.

While it was not discussed in the previous lesson, the parotid gland is not mixed. Its salivary product is entirely serous.

The sublingual caruncle (from the submandibular gland) and the sublingual duct openings (from the sublingual gland) are the intraoral openings allowing for the egress of saliva from the glands.

"*The*" Floor of the Mouth: The Mylohyoid Muscle

The mylohyoid muscle originates at the mylohyoid line of the mandible and inserts onto the midline raphe as well as the body of the hyoid bone. It acts to elevate both the hyoid bone and the tongue. It also depresses the mandible. The mylohyoid is efferently innervated by the mylohyoid nerve (a branch of the inferior alveolar nerve which is itself a branch of the mandibular division of the trigeminal nerve).

Like the anterior belly of the digastric muscle, the mylohyoid muscle is embryologically derived from the second pharyngeal arch. Both muscles, therefore, receive the same innervation (the nerve to the mylohyoid).

The mylohyoid muscle serves as the floor of the paralingual space intraorally (that space lateral and inferior to the tongue) as well as the roof of the submandibular space extraorally. In all practicality, the mylohyoid muscle is *the floor* of the mouth. The paralingual space is above it and the submandibular space is below it. The paralingual space is considered "intraoral" while the submandibular space is "extraoral". The dividing line between intraoral and extraoral is the mylohyoid muscle.

It should be noted that the hyoglossus muscle lies deep (internal) to the mylohyoid muscle. The hyoglossus originates from the hyoid bone and inserts into the substance of the tongue by intermingling with its intrinsic fibers. It acts to depress and retract the tongue and is efferently served by the hypoglossal nerve. It is considered an extrinsic muscle of the tongue and is an important landmark at the posterior aspect of the paralingual space. (1, Muscles of the Head and Neck - Hyoglossus)

When examining the floor of the mouth from an intraoral aspect one finds the geniohyoid muscle directly superior to the mylohyoid muscle. The geniohyoid muscle originates from the mental spines of the mandible and inserts into the body of the hyoid bone. It acts to elevate the hyoid bone and to depress the mandible. It is efferently innervated by C1 ventral primary ramus fibers traveling with the hypoglossal nerve. (2, Muscles of the Head and Neck - Geniohyoid)

It should be noted that the thyrohyoid and geniohyoid muscles are similar in that both receive ansa cervicalis fibers that travel with the hypoglossal nerve.

Tongue

The tongue is comprised of both extrinsic and intrinsic musculature.

The intrinsic muscles include the inferior and superior longitudinal muscles, the transverse muscles, and the vertical muscles. These are efferently served by the hypoglossal nerve. These muscles are very difficult to distinguish individually on most cadaveric specimens and essentially make up most of the bulk of the tongue proper.

The extrinsic muscles include the genioglossus, styloglossus, hyoglossus and palatoglossus muscles. Most all of the extrinsic muscles of the tongue are efferently innervated by the hypoglossal nerve. The only exception to this rule is palatoglossus which is innervated by the vagus nerve. This can be readily remembered as the vagus nerve innervates most of the musculature of the palate and pharynx.

The genioglossus muscle, like the geniohyoid, originates from the mental spine of the mandible. It inserts into the tongue and acts to protrude and depress the tongue. It is efferently innervated by the hypoglossal nerve like most other extrinsic muscles of the tongue. (3, Muscles of the Head and Neck - Genioglossus)

The styloid process has three muscles which originate from it. All are innervated by different efferent nerves. One, the stylohyoid was discussed earlier in this chapter. It is innervated by the facial nerve. Stylopharyngeus is a muscle of the posterior pharynx and will be discussed later in the book. It is served efferently be the glossopharyngeal nerve. Finally, the styloglossus is an extrinsic muscle of the tongue. It is served efferently by the hypoglossal nerve. (4, Muscles of the Head and Neck - Stylopharyngeus)

General sensation (afferent) to the anterior tongue is provided by the lingual nerve (from V3). General sensation to the posterior tongue is provided by the glossopharyngeal nerve (CN IX).

The sense of taste is carried from the anterior 2/3 of the tongue via the chorda tympani nerve (from CN VII). The sense of taste is carried from the posterior 1/3 of the tongue via the glossopharyngeal nerve (CN IX). There are also a small amount of scattered taste fibers from the vagus nerve (CN X) at the base of the tongue.

The tongue is given movement (efferent innervation) by means of the vagus nerve (as it serves the palatoglossus) and the hypoglossal nerve.

Tongue Vasculature

The lingual artery passes deep to the hyoglossus muscle before its arrival into the paralingual space. Recall that the lingual artery gives off the dorsal lingual artery at the posterior border of the hyoglossus and the deep lingual artery at the anterior border of the hyoglossus. The distal-most extension of the lingual artery is the sublingual artery serving the tip of the tongue.

Venous structures draining the tongue include the lingual, deep lingual, and sublingual veins. The vena comitans also drain the tongue base and travel alongside the hypoglossal nerve in the deepest recess of the paralingual space.

Paralingual Space

The paralingual space is bounded by the mandible (anterolaterally), tongue base (medially), and the mylohyoid and hyoglossus muscles (inferiorly). The oral mucosa comprises the roof of the paralingual space.

Within the paralingual space is the lingual nerve, hypoglossal nerve (with vena comitans), submandibular duct, and lingual artery (deep to the hyoglossus). The submandibular ganglion is also found within the paralingual space attached to the lingual nerve.

The lingual nerve is a branch of the mandibular division of the trigeminal nerve. It is carrying sensory information back to the brain from the oral cavity ("general afferent" information).

The chorda tympani nerve is a branch of the facial nerve carrying both autonomic preganglionic fibers to the submandibular ganglion as well as sensory information back to the brain from the tongue ("special afferent" information which is specifically taste from the anterior two-thirds of the tongue). The chorda tympani hitches a ride with the lingual nerve very soon after it (the chorda tympani) exits the skull via the petrotympanic fissure at the posterior aspect of the mandibular fossa.

The autonomic fibers from the facial nerve destined to innervate the submandibular and sublingual glands pass through the submandibular ganglion. Preganglionics intended for the sublingual glands synapse with postganglionics in the ganglion. Preganglionics intended for the submandibular gland merely pass through the ganglion and enter the glandular substance where they synapse locally ("within the gland") with their postganglionic counterparts.

The hypoglossal nerve is efferently serving musculature of the tongue. It commonly has multiple small veins (vena comitans) which travel with it to drain the region.

The submandibular duct empties its contents into the oral cavity inferior to the tip of the tongue via the sublingual caruncle. [Note: The sublingual glands are located along the anteromedial border of the mandible in the anterior most region of the paralingual space. They lie below the lingual nerve and submandibular duct and do not have any named ducts emptying into the oral cavity. Instead, they give off multiple unnamed ducts which pass directly through the oral mucosa lateral to the sublingual caruncle.]

A very important three dimensional relationship exists in the paralingual space between the lingual nerve and the submandibular duct. The lingual nerve is always deep (inferior) to the submandibular duct. The lingual nerve travels from the trunk of V3 (at the foramen ovale) along the medial border ("inner surface") of the mandible. It hugs the bone immediately lingual to the mandibular molar roots. It travels in this manner from a posterior to anterior direction. As it approaches the anterior aspect of the paralingual space it travels from lateral to medial below the submandibular duct. In this way the lingual nerve forms a "sling" holding the submandibular duct from below. The lingual nerve may be readily injured in procedures involving the mandibular molar roots given the close proximity between nerve and root.

The lingual artery is also in the paralingual space, but it is deep to the hyoglossus muscle. It is only visible after it emerges from below the muscle on its posterior to anterior course. It gives off the dorsal lingual artery at the posterior border of the hyoglossus and the deep lingual artery at the anterior border of the hyoglossus. The distal-most extension of the lingual artery is the sublingual artery serving the tip of the tongue.

The paralingual space is important clinically. Recall that the medial border of the mandible forms the lateral border of the paralingual space. In order to approach the space extraorally the clinician must pass through the sublingual and submental triangles. It may be more readily accessed from a superior approach intraorally by merely reflecting the roof of the paralingual space (the oral mucosa).

Take time to review the image of the paralingual space included at the end of this chapter. This image should be memorized and the student should label the image on his/her own. (Note: Image modeled after original art in Laboratory and Study Guide for Head and Neck Anatomy, 2013).

Fascial Space Pathology

Infections and other pathologies can set up shop within the various spaces of the head and neck including the submandibular space and the paralingual space. One particularly dangerous entity is called Ludwig's Angina.

As a brief introduction, Ludwig's Angina is a bacterial infection of the floor of the mouth inferior to the tongue base. It is technically a "cellulitis" which is caused by an uncontrolled bacterial infection of the paralingual space and the submandibular/submental triangles inferior to the mylohyoid muscle. The infection is bilateral and is very aggressive. Abscess formation is rare, and the lymphatic system is classically uninvolved.

Signs and symptoms of Ludwig's Angina include neck pain, neck swelling, redness of the neck, fever, weakness, fatigue, excessive tiredness, confusion or other mental status changes, and difficulty breathing (this final symptom indicates an emergency situation).

Treatment of Ludwig's Angina must be urgent if not emergent as airway maintenance is crucial. Airway maintenance typically includes either intubation or tracheotomy. The next major goal of treatment is eradication of the infection via intravenous antibiotics, dental treatment (to treat any infections, etc.), and surgery in order to evacuate the abscess. Prompt dental treatment of oral infections serves to prevent Ludwig's Angina. It is important to remember that the fascial spaces of the head and neck can intercommunicate with one another in certain pathologic circumstances. Therefore, infections in one space may move to other spaces of the head, neck, or thorax.

Sources Cited:

1-4. Gest, et al. Anatomy Tables (electronic MedCharts). Ann Arbor, MI. 2000

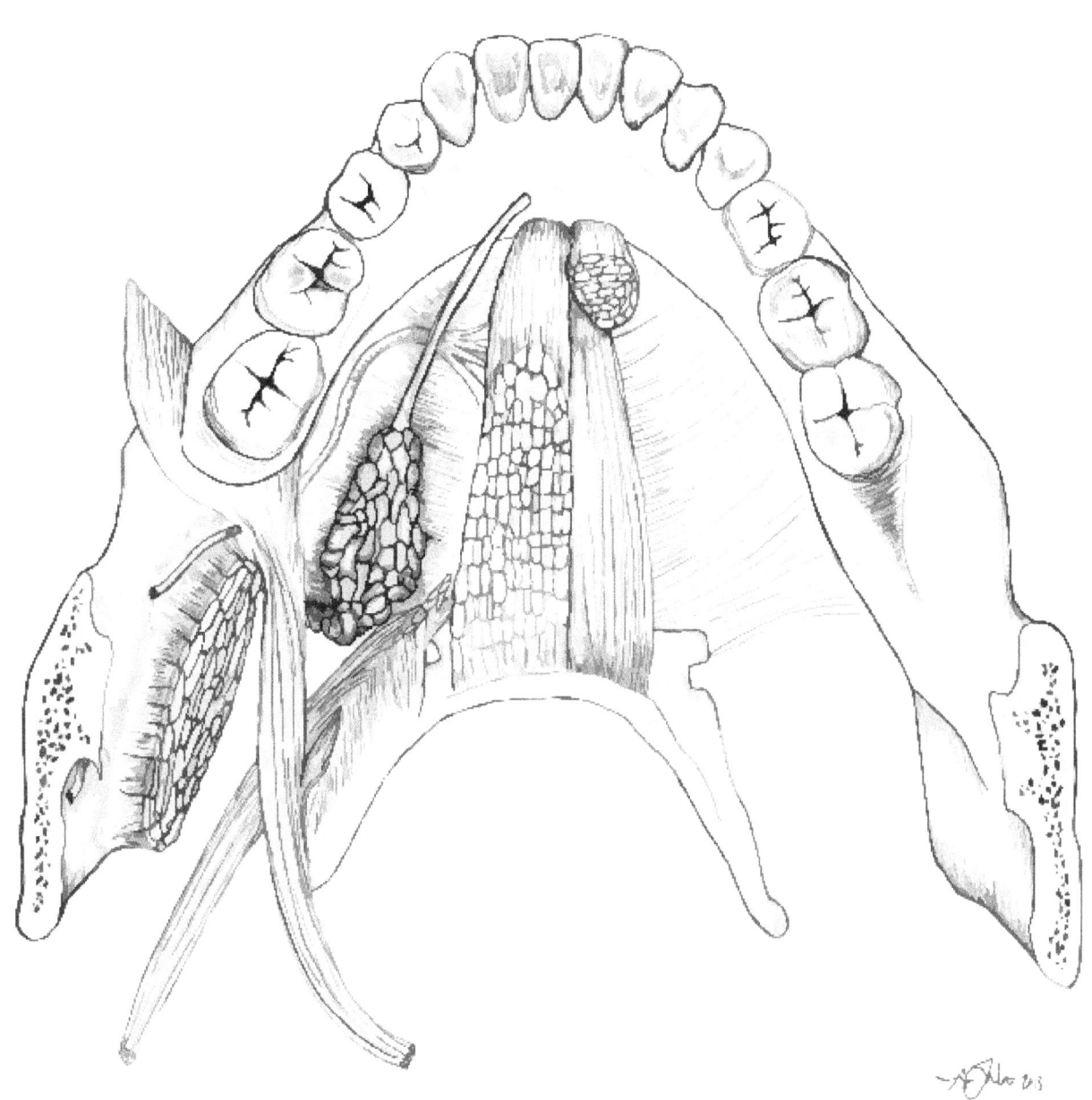

Laboratory Approach

☐1. Review the boundaries and contents of the submandibular and sublingual triangles.

☐2. Examine the boundaries of the paralingual space while identifying its contents and the relationships therein.

☐3. Examine the surface features of the tongue.

☐4. Examine the extrinsic and intrinsic musculature of the tongue as well as its neurovascular supply.

☐5. Examine the course of the facial and lingual arteries from the external carotid artery to their most distal branches.

☐6. Examine the floor of the mouth with special attention to the mylohyoid muscle, its neurovascular supply, and how the paralingual space (above) and submandibular space (below) are formed.

☐7. Examine the osteology of the mandible and hyoid bone with particular attention paid to the tongue base and intraoral muscle attachments.

Paralingual space & its contents
    Sublingual gland & ducts
    Submandibular gland (deep lobe) and duct
    Lingual n.
        chorda tympani
        submandibular ganglion
    Hypoglossal n. & its vena comitans
    Sublingual branch of the lingual a.
        Dorsal lingual branches
        Sublingual branch
        Deep lingual a.

Arteries
    Facial
        Ascending palatine br.
        Tonsillar br.
        Submental br.
    Lingual
        Dorsal lingual br.
        Sublingual br.
        Deep lingual

Muscles
    Anterior and Posterior Digastric (Bellies) mm.
    Mylohyoid
    Geniohyoid
    Extrinsic tongue mm.
        hyoglossus
        styloglossus
        genioglossus
    Intrinsic tongue mm.
        superior & inferior longitudinal mm.
        transversus
        verticalis

External Tongue
    Median lingual sulcus
    Filiform papillae
    Fungiform papillae
    Vallate papillae
    Sulcus terminalis
    Foramen cecum
    Lingual frenulum
    Fimbriated fold
    Epiglottis
    Valleculae epiglottica
    Median glossoepiglottic fold
    Lateral glossoepiglottic fold
    Sublingual fold

Openings of sublingual ducts
Sublingual caruncle

Osteology

TEMPORAL BONE

External aspect:
Squamous portion
External acoustic meatus
Jugular fossa
Tympanic portion
Mastoid process
Inferior tympanic canaliculus
Petrous portion
Mastoid foramen
Zygomatic process
Mastoid notch
Mandibular fossa
   Articular surface
   Non-articular surface
Petrotympanic fissure
Temporal line
Articular eminence
Carotid canal
Styloid process

Endocranial aspect:
Squamous portion
Petrous portion
Arcuate eminence
Sigmoid sinus sulcus
Superior petrosal pinus
Internal acoustic meatus
Mastoid foramen
Trigeminal fossa
Grooves for middle meningeal a.
Hiatus(es) for the greater & lesser petrosal nn.

Muscles of Mastication and the Temporomandibular Joint

<u>Introduction</u>

This lesson will study the temporomandibular joint, its related ligamentous structures, the mandible, and the muscles of mastication. The neurovasculature of the region will be introduced in this chapter, but will be formally studied in detail in the following chapter.

<u>Temporomandibular Joint (TMJ)</u>

As the name implies, the temporomandibular joint (TMJ) refers to the area of articulation between the condylar head of the mandible and the temporal bone of the skull base. The four major muscles of mastication will act at this joint allowing for chewing and other directed mandibular movements. The movements of the mandible are determined by the architecture of the TMJ, the actions of the muscles of mastication, and the contacts between the maxillary and mandibular teeth ("occlusion").

Take time at this point to study the mandible and its various bony landmarks as well as the bony anatomy of the skull base.

An inferior view of the external skull base reveals the mandibular fossa. The articular eminence and tubercle lie at the anterior border of the mandibular fossa and are specializations of the temporal bone. This is the site of direct articulation of the condylar head of the mandible with the temporal bone.

Take time to review other important landmarks of the external skull base which have been studied in previous chapters. Assimilate that knowledge with the location of the mandibular fossa. Visualize the articulation of the condylar head of the mandible at the articular tubercle.

Notice that the petrotympanic fissure can be found at the posterior portion of the mandibular fossa. It is through this bony opening that the chorda tympani passes. Recall that the chorda tympani is carrying both autonomic fibers (destined for the submandibular ganglion in the paralingual space) and taste fibers from the anterior two-thirds of the tongue.

Even though the petrotympanic fissure is perilously close to the condylar head of the mandible, it is protected from injury since the head of the condyle directly articulates at the articular tubercle medial and posterior to the zygomatic arch.

Of particular importance in this chapter are the condylar process (essentially the head and neck of the mandible) and the ramus. On the internal aspect of the ramus of the mandible can be found the mandibular foramen which allows for the transmission of the inferior alveolar nerve (branch of V3). The mandibular foramen can be found along a line passing between the region of greatest concavity on the anterior and posterior surfaces of the mandibular ramus. (1, p. 90)

The musculoskeletal complex of the TMJ is functionally unique in that there are two temporomandiblar joints connected via one bone (the mandible). Ergo, contraction of the muscles of mastication on one side results in movement bilaterally (to differing degrees).

It should be noted here that radiographically we see articulation between the posterior slope of the articular tubercle (of the temporal bone) and the condyle head of the mandible, NOT in the mandibular fossa. The mandibular fossa is very thin and cannot take the stress of direct articulation.

The TMJ is primarily composed of an articular capsule and a lateral ligament which is anterior and inferior to the capsule proper. The joint is stabilized via two other accessory ligaments: the sphenomandibular and stylomandibular ligaments. The sphenomandibular ligament passes from the skull base (spine of the sphenoid bone) to the region of bone directly inferior to the mandibular foramen and lingula. It fuses with the deep fascia found in the interpterygoid space which will be studied in the following lesson. The stylomandibular ligament passes between the styloid process and the posteroinferior border of the mandible.

Notice that the TMJ is immediately anterior to the external acoustic meatus. The posterior boundary of the joint is the postglenoid process, and the anterior boundary of the joint is the articular eminence of the zygomatic arch (its posterior root).

Muscles of Mastication

The muscles of mastication include the temporalis, the masseter, the medial pterygoid, and the lateral pterygoid muscles.

One of the muscles of mastication, the temporalis, originates within the temporal fossa at the lateral aspect of the skull. This fossa space is immediately lateral to the pterion and is formed by the frontal, parietal, sphenoid, and temporal bones.

The investing fascia of the temporalis muscle attaches to the superior temporal line while the muscle fibers themselves attach to the inferior temporal line. The temporalis muscle then inserts onto the coronoid process (after passing deep to the zygomatic arch) and anterior surface of the ramus of the mandible. It acts to elevate and retract the mandible.

The nervous supply to the temporalis muscle is provided by the anterior and posterior deep temporal nerves, small branches of V3 which enter the deep surface of temporalis.

Deep and anterior to the TMJ resides the infratemporal fossa where the mandibular branches of the trigeminal nerve arise from the foramen ovale. This region will be studied in detail in the following chapter. At this point it is important to know that the infratemporal fossa is the eruption point of V3.

The boundaries of the infratemporal fossa are (2, Dissector Answers - Infratemporal Fossa and Oral Cavity):
>Medial: Lateral pterygoid plate
>Lateral: Medial surface of the ramus of the mandible
>Anterior: Tuberosity of the maxilla
>Posterior: Deep part of the parotid region
>Superior: Base of the skull (greater wing of sphenoid bone)
>Inferior: Medial pterygoid muscle

The contents of the infratemporal fossa are (3, Dissector Answers - Infratemporal Fossa and Oral Cavity):

  Medial pterygoid muscle
  Lateral pterygoid muscle
  Maxillary artery and vein
  Pterygoid plexus of veins
  Mandibular division of trigeminal nerve
  Otic ganglion

The masseter originates from the zygomatic arch and zygoma while inserting onto the lateral surface of the ramus (all the way inferior to the mandibular angle). It acts to elevate the mandible and is efferently served by the "nerve to the masseter", a branch of V3.

As an overarching concept, it is important to note that all of the muscles of mastication are supplied with blood via branches of the maxillary artery, and all of the muscles of mastication are efferently innervated by branches of the mandibular division of the trigeminal nerve.

The masseter and temporalis are powerful muscles of mastication.

The medial pterygoid muscle arises from the medial surface of the lateral pterygoid plate (as well as from the palatine and maxillary bones). It inserts onto the medial surface of the ramus of the mandible (and travels as inferior as the angle of the mandible). It acts to elevate and protract the mandible. It is efferently served by the medial pterygoid branch of the mandibular division of the trigeminal nerve. It is important to note that its actions mirror that of the masseter muscle. Its fiber direction is the same as that of the masseter and both muscles create a "sling" around the ramus and angle of the mandible.

The lateral pterygoid has two heads. The superior head takes origination from the greater wing of the sphenoid. The inferior head takes origination from the lateral surface of the lateral pterygoid plate. The superior head inserts into the capsule and articular disc of the TMJ while the inferior head inserts onto the neck of the mandible (at the pterygoid fovea). These muscles act to open the mouth. They are the only muscles of mastication to open the mouth. They are efferently innervated by the lateral pterygoid branch of the mandibular division of the trigeminal nerve.

It is very important to take extra time to memorize and understand the anatomy of the lateral pterygoid muscle. It is unique in multiple ways. It opens the mouth and also has two heads, one of which (the superior) attaches to the articular disc and moves it anteriorly past the articular eminence in opening movements of the mandible. Both heads of the lateral pterygoid must be functioning properly in order to have proper mouth opening. The inferior head moves the condylar apparatus while the superior head ensures that the disc is moving with the condylar head.

The mandibular division of the trigeminal nerve is typically found between the bellies of the medial and lateral pterygoid muscles. The maxillary artery (which supplies both muscles) is found between the muscles 50% of the time, and lateral to the lateral pterygoid muscle 50% of the time.

Note that there is an interpterygoid fascia between the medial and lateral pterygoid muscles. This will be studied in more detail in future chapters, but now it is important to note that it serves to allow freedom of movement between the muscles. Neurovascular structures also run through this fascia (i.e. one should notice V3 passing through the fascial plane as the inferior alveolar nerve makes its way to the mandibular foramen on the medial surface of the mandible).

The maxillary artery gives off branches which supply all of the muscles of mastication. Branches include the deep temporal arteries, the masseteric arteries, and the pterygoid arteries. Recall that the maxillary artery is a terminal branch of the external carotid artery arising deep and medial to the ramus of the mandible in the infratemporal fossa space. The superficial temporal artery is the other terminal branch of the external carotid artery. The superficial temporal artery also supplies structures in the TMJ region, including the joint itself.

Fascial Spaces

The masticator space can be subdivided into four smaller spaces: the superficial, intermediate, arthro-osseous, and deep.

Recall that every muscle in the human body is invested with fascia individually and that this fascia can extend and cover other structures within the region. In this particular case, the masticator fascia is covering all four muscles of mastication individually and is also creating a grouped compartment.

The superficial space is surrounding the temporalis and masseter muscles. The intermediate space is surrounding the lateral pterygoid muscle and the deep space is surrounding the medial pterygoid muscle.

The lateral pharyngeal space is medial to the masticator space and lateral to the pharyngeal wall and the constrictors.

The prevertebral space is posterior and deep to the pharyngeal spaces.

It is important to realize that there is continuity between these spaces. This is clinically important in assessing, treating, and tracking infectious processes in the head and neck, for example.

TMJ Summary

Articulation at the joint is between the temporal bone (zygomatic process --> the posterior slope of the articular tubercle/eminence defines the anterior boundary of the glenoid fossa) and mandible (the condylar head is 20mm by 10mm) with overlying hyaline cartilage on the bony surfaces under the age of 20 and fibrocartilage over compact bone in adults.

It should be noted that a thin layer of proliferative tissue exists over the fibrocartilage that allows remodeling (in functional change, wear, and tooth movement). Radiographically we see articulation between the posterior slope of the articular tubercle and the condyle, but NOT in the fossa (fossa is very thin and cannot take stress).

The TMJ capsule is comprised of dense collagenous fibers which span from temporal bone to disc to mandible.

In between the bones and within the capsule is the fibrous articular disc (biconcave) separating the joint space into two synovial cavities (compartments). The disc is thickest at the periphery and thinnest at stress-bearing regions. It merges with the surrounding capsule anteriorly (medially and laterally the disc and capsule attach to the condylar margins which necessitates movement of the condyle with the disc). The disc is connected posteriorly to the highly vascular connective tissue known as retrodiscal tissue.

The superior compartment is larger than the inferior compartment and permits freedom of movement between the disc and the articular eminence. Fibers of the lateral pterygoid muscle insert onto the anterior portion of the capsule and the articular disc (the discal fibers fuse with the fibers of the joint capsule itself).The inferior compartment is smaller and prohibits movement between the articular disc and the eminence.

Vascularization of the TMJ is accomplished by branches of the superficial temporal artery and maxillary artery. Articular structures are avascular and are supplied by synovial fluid (diffusion of nutrients). The disc periphery is very vascular, but its central region is avascular (it is supplied by peripheral vascularization and diffusion).

The innervation of the TMJ is accomplished via rich capsular innervation from the mandibular division of the trigeminal nerve with specific supply from the auriculotemporal nerve and also with branches from the masseteric nerve.

Clinically the TMJ is very important and is affected by many local and systemic pathologies including osteo and rheumatoid arthritis. Any disruption to the stomatognathic system (teeth, periodontal ligaments, alveolar bone, muscles of mastication, or the TMJ itself) may lead to temporomandibular disease (TMD) and is caused by changes in free-way dimensions (typically 2-4 mm) of the rest position from occlusal change, disease, muscle/nervous disorders, prostheses, etc.

The clinical manifestations mimic those of joint, muscular, or non-dental pain. Essentially, TMD is a subclassification of musculoskeletal disease.

There are many signs and symptoms of TMD. Crepitus (clicking) is very common and is likely from a delay in the anterior disc movement on opening and/or closing (snapping of the disc between the articular eminence and condyle). Dislocation of the mandible (can only happen in an anterior direction) can occur as the condyles slide down unchecked along the slope of articular eminence to pass anteriorly into the infratemporal fossa. This can be from spasm of the lateral pterygoids causing excessive contraction (such as in a long dental procedure), a yawn, or the indulgence in a triple-decker cheeseburger.

In fractures of the mandible (from trauma, a fall, etc.) care needs to be taken to avoid damage to CN VII and CN V since damage to V (particularly the auriculotemporal nerve) may lead to instability of the TMJ and subsequent TMD.

Sources Cited:

1. Brzezinski, et al. Laboratory and Study Guide for Head and Neck Anatomy: Dissection of the Head and Neck. Ann Arbor, MI. 2013

2-3. Dissector Answers - Infratemporal Fossa and Oral Cavity. 2000. http://www.med.umich.edu/lrc/coursepages/m1/anatomy2010/html/nervous_system/infratemp_ans.html

Laboratory Approach

☐1. Examine the temporal and infratemporal fossae.

☐2. Examine the muscles of mastication, their attachments, and their neurovascular supply.

☐3. Examine the temporomandibular joint, its component parts and its accessory ligaments.

☐4. Review the actions of the muscles of mastication and how contraction leads to opening and closing of the mandible.

<u>Key Regional Structures</u>

Temporomandibular joint (TMJ)
    Lateral ligament
    Articular capsule
    Upper & lower synovial cavities
    Synovial membranes
    Articular disc
    Sphenomandibular ligament
    Stylomandibular ligament
    Retrodiscal pad

Muscles of mastication
    Masseter
        superficial & deep portions
    Temporalis
    Lateral pterygoid
        superior (sphenomeniscus) head
        inferior head
    Medial pterygoid

Fascia
    Muscular fascia (including Temporal fascia)
    Interpterygoid fascia

Vasculature to the muscles of mastication (from external carotid a.)

Nerves to the muscles of mastication (from V3)

SPHENOID BONE

Body
Clivus
Tuberculum sellae
Carotid sulcus
Sella turcica
Dorsum sellae
Sphenoid sinus
Hypophyseal fossa
Posterior clinoid process

Lesser wing
Anterior clinoid process
Superior orbital fissure
Optic canal

Greater wing
Cerebral surface
Foramen spinosum
Infratemporal crest
Temporal surface
Foramen rotundum
Sphenoidal spine
Orbital surface
Foramen ovale

Pterygoid process
Pterygoid hamulus
Pterygoid fossa
Pterygoid canal
Lateral pterygoid plate
Medial pterygoid plate
Scaphoid fossa

Deep Face and the Infratemporal Fossa

Introduction

This chapter will review the neurovasculature of the TMJ region, as well as the structures contained within the infratemporal fossa.

The infratemporal fossa is a space deep to the ramus of the mandible and inferior to the skull base. It is deep and anterior to the TMJ. Once the condylar apparatus and ramus of the mandible have been removed, the infratemporal fossa space can be readily visualized.

The boundaries of the infratemporal fossa are: (1, Dissector Answers - Infratemporal Fossa and Oral Cavity):

      Medial: Lateral pterygoid plate
      Lateral: Medial surface of the ramus of the mandible
      Anterior: Tuberosity of the maxilla
      Posterior: Deep part of the parotid region
      Superior: Base of the skull (greater wing of sphenoid bone)
      Inferior: Medial pterygoid muscle

The contents of the infratemporal fossa are: (2, Dissector Answers - Infratemporal Fossa and Oral Cavity):

      Medial pterygoid muscle
      Lateral pterygoid muscle
      Maxillary artery and vein
      Pterygoid plexus of veins
      Mandibular division of trigeminal nerve
      Otic ganglion

Very importantly, the infratemporal fossa is where the mandibular branches of the trigeminal nerve arise from the foramen ovale. The maxillary artery and vein also reside within this fossa space, as do the pterygoid muscles.

Pterygoid Muscles

The medial and lateral pterygoids reside within the infratemporal fossa space, and the mandibular division of the trigeminal nerve typically passes between them in the pterygomandibular space.

Recall from the last lesson that the medial pterygoid muscle arises from the medial surface of the lateral pterygoid plate (as well as from the palatine and maxillary bones). It inserts onto the medial surface of the ramus of the mandible (and travels as inferior as the angle of the mandible). It acts to elevate and protract the mandible. It is efferently served by the medial pterygoid branch of the mandibular division of the trigeminal nerve. (3, Muscles of the Head and Neck - Medial Pterygoid)

The lateral pterygoid has two heads. The superior head takes origination from the greater wing of the sphenoid. The inferior head takes origination from the lateral surface of the lateral pterygoid plate. The superior head inserts into the capsule and articular disc of the TMJ, while the inferior head inserts onto the neck of the mandible. These muscles act to open the mouth. They are the only muscles of mastication to open the mouth. They are efferently innervated by the lateral pterygoid branch of the mandibular division of the trigeminal nerve. (4, Muscles of the Head and Neck - Lateral Pterygoid)

Examine the pterygoid fossae and scaphoid fossae on the external aspect of a skull base. These regions are part of the sphenoid bone.

The pterygoid fossa contains fibers of the medial pterygoid muscle, but the medial pterygoid's primary origination is from the medial aspect of the lateral pterygoid plate.

The pterygoid fossa and scaphoid fossa are better known as the attachment point of the tensor veli palatini muscle of the soft palate. This muscle, as well as the levator veli palatini of the soft palate will be studied in more detail in a later chapter.

Note that there is a mirror relationship of the masseter and medial pterygoid muscles as they create a sling around the mandibular ramus.

The temporalis is superior to the masseteropterygoid sling, and the lateral pterygoid is superior to it as well.

Recall also that there is an interpterygoid fascia between the medial and lateral pterygoid muscles. It is important to note that this fascia serves to allow freedom of movement between the muscles. Neurovascular structures also run through this fascia (i.e. one should notice V3 passing through the fascial plane as the inferior alveolar nerve makes its way to the mandibular foramen on the medial surface of the mandible).

Trigeminal Nerve (CN V) Review

The trigeminal nerve is divided into three primary divisions: the ophthalmic (V1), the maxillary (V2), and the mandibular (V3).

The V1 and V2 divisions are strictly afferent nerves ("general sensory afferents" or GSA). They only serve to bring back important sensory information to the central nervous system. They will be studied in detail later in this book.

The V3 division serves an afferent role to the face, but it also serves as the sole supplier of efferent fibers to the muscles of mastication. It also supplies two smaller muscles (the tensor tympani in the middle ear and the tensor veli palatini of the soft palate) which will be studied later in this book as well as the anterior belly of the digastric muscle and the mylohyoid muscle.

Since the fibers of the trigeminal nerve serve a wide area of cutaneous tissues, they also serve as "nervous super-highways" whereby autonomic nerves hitch a ride in order to safely arrive at their various destinations.

The trigeminal nerve starts as a single nerve as it arises from the pons. Very soon, however, it separates into its three primary divisions. This separation occurs before the divisions leave the cranial vault. The motor root (efferent) and trigeminal ganglion (afferent) regions of the trigeminal nerve can be found just proximal to the divisional separations.

While specifics relating to the motor root and trigeminal ganglion are discussed in more detail in other resources, it is important to know here that the motor root ultimately derives from the lateral midpontine tegmentum. It innervates the muscles of mastication, the tensors (of the middle ear and soft palate), the mylohyoid muscle, and the anterior belly of the digastric. The sensory portion (afferent innervation from the trigeminal ganglion) supplies the face, the mucous membranes of the nasal and oral cavities, the palate, the deep musculature of the face (proprioception), the TMJ, and the dura of the anterior and middle cranial fossae.

At this point, one should review the cutaneous (afferent) branches of the trigeminal nerve as well as the various openings and foramina of the skull base (including those which allow transmission of the trigeminal nerve divisions.

V1 will pass through the superior orbital fissure and innervate orbital, midface, and forehead structures.

V2 will pass through foramen rotundum and innervate midface structures (such as the posteroinferior aspect of the nasal cavity and nasopharynx and palate) and the maxillary teeth.

V3 will pass through foramen ovale and will innervate oral and mandibular structures and the mandibular teeth.

Arterial Supply of the Infratemporal Fossa

The maxillary artery (a terminal branch of the external carotid artery) resides within the infratemporal fossa. The maxillary artery serves all of the muscles of mastication, the TMJ, as well as deep midface structures (via the sphenopalatine artery) which will be studied in a later chapter.

One of the first superior branches of the maxillary artery is the middle meningeal artery which eventually serves the linings of the brain after passing through the foramen spinosum.

One of the first inferior branches of the maxillary artery is the inferior alveolar artery which travels with the inferior alveolar nerve through the mandibular foramen to serve the mandible.

Smaller distal branches of the maxillary artery serve the buccal aspect of the midface as well as the hard and soft palates.

Pterygomaxillary Fissure and Pterygopalatine Fossa

The pterygomaxillary fissure is the lateral entrance into the pterygopalatine fossa. This fissure and fossa are important because they are where V2 and the pterygopalatine ganglion can be found.

The lateral wall of the pterygopalatine fossa contains the pterygomaxillary fissure (between the lateral pterygoid plate and the maxillary tuberosity).

The medial wall of the pterygopalatine fossa contains the sphenopalatine foramen. This foramen is the lateral entry into the nasal cavity (and allows passage of branches of V2 which will serve the nasal cavity as well as branches of the sphenopalatine artery which will also serve the nasal cavity).

Autonomic Nerves

At this point the student has studied the otic ganglion and the submandibular ganglion. These ganglia are associated with the glossopharyngeal and facial nerves (respectively). Review these two ganglia and their role in autonomic innervation to the salivary glands.

The pterygopalatine ganglia (within the pterygopalatine fossa) will now be studied. This ganglia is associated with fibers of the facial nerve which serve to supply postganglionic parasympathetic fibers to the entire midface and lacrimal gland of the orbit.

Preganglionic autonomic fibers from CN VII leave the facial nerve while it is still superior to the middle and inner ear spaces. These fibers are bundled as the greater petrosal nerve.

The greater petrosal nerve leaves temporal bone via the hiatus for the greater petrosal nerve (which is located medially to the hiatus for the lesser petrosal nerve) on the petrous ridge of the temporal bone. It then passes over the skull base until it arrives at the foramen lacerum through which it will exit.

Upon its exit, the greater petrosal nerve joins the deep petrosal nerve (postganglionic sympathetic fibers from the superior cervical ganglion) to become the nerve of the pterygoid canal.

The preganglionic parasympathetic fibers of the greater petrosal nerve bundled with postganglionic sympathetics of the deep petrosal nerve travel as the newly formed nerve of the pterygoid canal to the posterior wall of the pterygopalatine fossa where they encounter the pterygopalatine ganglia.

At the pterygopalatine ganglia the preganglionic parasympathetic fibers synapse (within the ganglia) with their postsynaptic counterparts. [Note: The postganglionic sympathetic fibers merely pass through the ganglia having already synapsed in the superior cervical ganglia in the neck.]

The postganglionic parasympathetic fibers of CN VII ultimately provide secretomotor innervation (efferently) to the lacrimal gland and glands of the midface region (nasal cavity, maxillary sinus, and the palate).

Veins of the Lateral and Deep Face

The superficial temporal vein lies at the superoposterior aspect of the face directly anterior to the external ear. It drains inferiorly into the retromandibular vein.

The retromandibular vein then divides into an anterior and posterior branch. The anterior branch joins with the facial and lingual veins to create the common venous trunk which drains into the internal jugular vein. The posterior branch joins with the posterior auricular vein to create the external jugular vein which passes inferiorly over the sternocleidomastoid muscle before draining into the subclavian vein.

Note that deep veins of the face such as the pterygoid veins and maxillary veins communicate with the dural venous sinuses and the retromandibular veins. As such, they ultimately drain into the jugular or subclavian veins. These deep facial veins communicate with the cavernous sinus. This is clinically important in cases of cellulits or facial lacerations which become infected. In these cases the pathogens (typically bacterial in nature) can pass through the deep facial veins and access the cavernous sinus space. Infections in the cavernous sinus are particularly dangerous as they can compromise the wall of the internal carotid artery (which passes through the cavernous sinus) leading to hemorrhagic stroke.

Sources Cited:

1-2. Dissector Answers - Infratemporal Fossa and Oral Cavity. 2000.
http://www.med.umich.edu/lrc/coursepages/m1/anatomy2010/html/nervous_system/infratemp_ans.html

3-4. Gest, et al. Anatomy Tables (electronic MedCharts). Ann Arbor, MI. 2000

Laboratory Approach

☐1. Examine the infratemporal fossa and describe its boundaries and contents.

☐2. Review and examine the muscles of mastication, their attachments, and their neurovascular supply.

☐3. Examine the interpterygoid fascia and its bony attachments.

☐4. Examine the mandibular division of the trigeminal nerve from its arrival within the infratemporal fossa to all branches within the facial region.

☐5. Examine the maxillary artery from its arrival within the infratemporal fossa to its various branches (focusing on the first and second parts of the maxillary artery).

☐6. Examine the pterygoid plexus of veins and the various interconnections with other regional venous structures.

☐7. Examine the mandible and muscles of mastication in relationship to the infratemporal fossa.

Key Regional Structures

Mandibular division of the trigeminal nerve
    Branches of the trunk
        Meningeal n.
        Medial pterygoid n.
        Tensor veli palatini n.
        Tensor tympani n.
    Anterior division
        Masseteric n.
        Posterior deep temporal n.
        Buccal n.
          Anterior deep temporal n.
        Lateral pterygoid n.
    Posterior division
        Lingual n.
        Inferior alveolar n.
          Mylohyoid n.
          Mental n.
        Auriculotemporal n.

Regional autonomic nerves
        Otic ganglion
        Submandibular ganglion
        Chorda tympani

Maxillary artery
    First part
        Deep auricular branch
        Anterior tympanic branch
        Middle & accessory meningeal aa.
        Inferior alveolar a.
    Second part
        Deep temporal branches
        Pterygoid branches
        Masseteric a.
        Buccal a.

Pterygoid plexus of veins

Pharynx and the Larynx

<u>Introduction</u>

This chapter will study the pharyngeal and laryngeal regions.

<u>Pharynx Overview</u>

The pharynx is essentially the region posterior to the nasal, oral, and laryngeal cavities. The region most posterior to the nasal cavity is the nasopharynx. The region most posterior to the oral cavity is the oropharynx. The region most posterior to the laryngeal cavity is the laryngopharynx.

The pharynx is that common area which allows the passage of air and food on its way to the trachea and esophagus, respectively.

The pharyngeal wall is composed of three constrictor muscles. These three muscles are stacked within one another (liked stacked cups). The inferior-most fibers of the superior constrictor are found deep to ("within the tube created by") the middle constrictor's superior-most fibers. The inferior-most fibers of the middle constrictor are found deep to ("within the tube created by") the inferior constrictor's superior-most fibers.

The larynx represents the superior-most aspect of the airway. It is immediately anterior to the laryngopharynx and is comprised of the epiglottic, cricoid and thyroid cartilages along with the vocal apparatus within this cartilaginous skeleton (arytenoid cartilage, various ligaments, and muscles of speech). The so-called laryngoskeleton is comprised of the cricoid, thyroid, arytenoid, and epiglottic complex. Intrinsic muscles of the larynx are found within this skeleton (and produce speech) and extrinsic muscles are found outside of this skeleton (and attach the laryngoskeleton to other musculoskeletal attachment points).

The larynx functions to produce speech and control the flow of air into and out of the lower airways.

The posterior wall of the pharynx is immediately anterior to the vertebral column and is invested in visceral fascia (a.k.a. buccopharyngeal fascia as it overlies the pharynx). The vertebral column is invested in prevertebral fascia.

Recall the "danger space", which is located between the visceral fascia and the prevertebral fascia. This space does not actually exist in reality since the two fascial boundaries essentially make contact with each other. It is a potential space filled with loose connective tissue. In cases of pathology, however, this space can "open up" allowing for infections, tumors, and other entities to take up residence.

This "danger space" extends from the skull base all the way inferiorly to the mediastinum in the thorax. It is along this highway that any oral pathology may spread into the thorax.

When a line is drawn from the junction of the hard and soft palates superiorly (the so-called "vibrating line") through the posterior lamina of the cricoid ring inferiorly, two regions are created. The anterior regions are referred to as "cavities". They include the oral cavity, the nasal cavity, and the larynx. The posterior regions are referred to as pharyngeal spaces. They include the nasopharynx, the oropharynx, and the laryngopharynx. The nasopharynx is that pharyngeal region superior to the palate and posterior to the nasal cavity. The oropharynx is that pharyngeal region inferior to the palate, superior to the hyoid bone and posterior to the oral cavity. The laryngopharynx is that pharyngeal region posterior to the larynx between the cricoid ring and the hyoid bone.

Within the nasopharynx can be found the torus ("cushion") and ostium ("opening") of the auditory tube. The auditory tube (a.k.a. Eustachian tube) connects the middle ear with the nasopharynx so that pressure can be equilibrated across the tympanic membrane (a.k.a. "ear drum"). The contents of the middle ear and nasopharynx will be studied in subsequent lessons.

Within the oropharynx can be found the palatine tonsils. These tonsils are located between the palatoglossal and palatopharyngeal folds. These folds are created by the oral mucosa which overlies the palatoglossus and palatopharyngeus muscles. These two muscles both originate from the palatine aponeurosis. One inserts into the tongue (palatoglossus) while the other inserts into the posterior wall of the pharynx (palatopharyngeus). Both muscles elevate that which they insert into, and both are efferently served by the vagus nerve (CN X).

It should be noted that the term "fold" in gross anatomy typically refers to the mucosal lining which overlies deeper structures.

Pharyngeal Constrictors

Review the inferior aspect of the external skull base. The constrictors attach to the skull base at the pharyngeal tubercle (occipital bone) via the pharyngeal raphae.

The superior constrictor originates from the medial pterygoid plate, the pterygoid hamulus, the pterygomandibular raphe, and the mylohyoid line of the mandible. It inserts into the pharyngeal tubercle and the midline pharyngeal raphe. It acts to constrict the pharynx and is efferently served by the vagus nerve. (1, Muscles of the Head and Neck - Superior Pharyngeal Constrictor)

The small region between the superior-most fibers of the superior pharyngeal constrictor and the skull base is occupied by a layer of fascial sheets. The outermost sheet is the buccopharyngeal fascia and the innermost sheet is the pharyngobasilar fascia. These two fascial sheets are in contact with one another and aid in the anchoring of the superior constrictor fibers to the skull base.

The line of demarcation between the superior and middle pharyngeal constrictors is created by the insertion of the stylopharyngeus muscle. This muscle originates from the styloid process and inserts into the pharyngeal wall and thyroid cartilage. It acts to elevate the larynx and is efferently innervated by the glossopharyngeal nerve. This is very important since it is the only muscle efferently innervated by the glossopharyngeal nerve. The major role of the glossopharyngeal nerve is that of afferent supply to the pharynx. (2, Muscles of the Head and Neck - Stylopharyngeus)

The middle pharyngeal constrictor originates from the greater and lesser horns of the hyoid bone and the inferior aspect of the stylohyoid ligament. It inserts into the midline pharyngeal raphe and is efferently innervated by the vagus nerve. It acts to constrict the pharynx. (3, Muscles of the Head and Neck - Middle Pharyngeal Constrictor)

The inferior pharyngeal constrictor originates from the oblique line of the thyroid cartilage and the lateral aspect of the cricoid ring. It inserts into the midline pharyngeal raphe and is efferently innervated by the vagus nerve. It acts to constrict the pharynx. (4, Muscles of the Head and Neck - Inferior Pharyngeal Constrictor)

In general, the superior constrictor originates from sphenoid and mandibular bony attachment points. The middle constrictor originates from hyoid bony attachments, and the inferior constrictors originate from the laryngeal skeleton (cricoid and thyroid cartilages). As an overarching point, the musculature of the pharynx is primarily skeletal muscle and arises embryologically from mesenchymal tissue of the fourth pharyngeal arch.

All three constrictors of the pharynx are arterially supplied by the ascending pharyngeal artery and the inferior constrictor is additionally supplied by the superior and inferior thyroid arteries. The pharynx is drained via the pharyngeal plexus of veins which ultimately drains into the internal jugular vein. This pharyngeal plexus also communicates with the pterygoid venous plexus.

Pharyngeal Innervation

All of the efferent innervation of the pharynx is supplied by the vagus nerve with the exception of the stylopharyngeus muscle which is supplied by the glossopharyngeal nerve.

The afferent innervation, by contrast, is regional in nature. The nasopharynx is supplied by V2, the oropharynx is supplied by the glossopharyngeal nerve, and the laryngopharynx is supplied by the vagus nerve.

The pharyngeal plexus of nerves can be found overlying the inferior portion of the posterior pharynx. It is essentially the intermingling of afferent and efferent nerve fibers in the region (glossopharyngeal and vagal fibers, respectively). It also contains vasomotor innervation from the superior cervical sympathetic ganglion which will innervate vascular smooth muscle.

Soft Palate Musculature

The veli palatini muscles will be studied in detail in layers here and elsewhere in this book. They are introduced here since they are readily encountered as one studies the naso and oropharyngeal regions.

The inferior layer of the soft palate is formed by the tensor veli palatini muscle.

The tensor veli palatini originates from the scaphoid fossa (sphenoid bone) and the lateral wall of the auditory tube cartilage. It inserts into the palatine aponeurosis after passing around the hamular hook of the medial pterygoid plate. It acts to tense the soft palate (thus its name) and open the auditory tube. It is served by V3 and the ascending pharyngeal artery. (5, Muscles of the Head and Neck - Tensor Veli Palatini)

All palatal muscles are innervated efferently by the vagus nerve except the tensor veli palatini which is served by V3.

The tensor veli palatini muscle's primary job is to keep the soft palate taut and to open the auditory tube.

Note that the superior pharyngeal constrictor is forming the superior posterior pharynx. It passes anteriorly to attach to the pterygomandibular raphe where it meets the buccinator muscle fibers passing posteriorly.

Superior to the tensor veli palatini is the levator veli palatini muscle.

The levator veli palatini originates from the apex of the petrous portion of the temporal bone and the medial wall of the auditory tube cartilage. It inserts into the musculature and fascia of the soft palate as well as the palatine aponeurosis. It acts to elevate the soft palate (thus its name) and is served by the vagus nerve and the ascending pharyngeal artery. (6, Muscles of the Head and Neck - Levator Veli Palatini)

The superiormost muscle of the soft palate is the palatopharyngeus. It originates from the bony palate and inserts into the posterior wall of the pharynx and the posterior margin of the thyroid cartilage. It acts to elevate the larynx and is served by the vagus nerve and the ascending pharyngeal artery. (7, Muscles of the Head and Neck - Palatopharyngeus)

Larynx Overview

The larynx is found in the anterior and deep neck. It is covered superficially by the infrahyoid muscles and the thyroid gland. It is essentially the "voice box".

The laryngeal inlet is protected by the epiglottis during deglutition.

Note that the hyoid bone is found at the C3-C4 vertebral level, and that the cricoid ring is found at the C5-C6 vertebral level. These two structures denote the superior and inferiormost extents of the larynx, respectively. The larynx, therefore, sits between the C3 and C6 vertebral levels. The hyoid bone marks the superiormost extent of the laryngoskeleton and the cricoid ring marks the inferiormost extent of the laryngoskeleton. Arytenoid, thyroid, and epiglottic cartilages are found between these two landmarks.

The thyrohyoid membrane is between the hyoid bone and the thyroid cartilage. Small neurovascular structures pass through this membrane to serve the upper larynx.

The cricothyroid membrane is between the thyroid and cricoid cartilages. The vocal cords are superior to this membrane, and it is through this membrane that one performs emergency airway maneuvers.

On the superior portion of the posterior lamina of the cricoid ring are the arytenoid cartilages. Notice that the vocal ligaments pass from the vocal processes of the arytenoid cartilages to the inside surface of the thyroid cartilage lamina. Musculature and mucosa cover these vocal ligaments creating the true vocal folds, which the lay population refers to as the "vocal cords".

Recall that the only complete ring in the airway is the cricoid ring. The tracheal rings are not complete, but are open posteriorly.

Small apertures ("openings") at the posterolateral aspect of the thyrohyoid membrane allow for the passage of neurovascular structures into and out of the larynx. These neurovascular structures penetrating the thyrohyoid membrane are the superior laryngeal artery (a branch of the superior thyroid artery) and the internal branch of the superior laryngeal nerve (a branch of the vagus nerve). This neurovasculature serves the superior internal aspect of the larynx. The internal branch of the superior laryngeal nerve afferently innervates all of the laryngeal mucosa superior to the vocal folds.

The arytenoid cartilages may be seen articulating with the posterior lamina of the cricoid ring.

The median cricothyroid ligament may be visualized from a lateral approach. This ligament arises from the cricoid ring and attaches to the thyroid cartilage anteriorly. It also attaches laterally into the vocal ligament.

While it is challenging to visualize in two-dimensional images, the cricothyroid ligament is essentially creating a "cone shape". The bottom (and widest aspect) of the cone is the origination of the ligament from the cricoid ring. The top of the cone is the insertion of the ligament into the vocal ligaments. It is reasonable and accurate to consider the superior "free edge" of the cricothyroid ligament to be continuous with the vocal ligament.

A membrane of connective tissue passes from the lateral and inferior borders of the epiglottis and attaches to the inner surface of the thyroid cartilage (superior to the attachment point of the vocal ligament) and the superior aspect of the arytenoid cartilage (superior to the attachment point of the vocal ligament). The inferior "free edge" which is created is called the vestibular ligament or the false vocal cord. It is called the false vocal fold when it is covered with mucosa. This entire membrane is called the quadrangular membrane and creates an upside-down cone (which is wider at the top and narrower at the bottom).

The space between the false vocal folds is called the rima vestibuli and the space between the true vocal folds is called the rima glottidis.

The vocal ligaments (and true vocal folds) move from side to side via actions of the laryngeal musculature which attaches to the arytenoid cartilage and moves it at its articulation with the cricoid ring.

The space above the false vocal folds is called the vestibular space (or vestibule).

The space between the true and false vocal folds is called the laryngeal ventricle.

Laryngeal Musculature

There are many small muscles which assist in the movement of the true vocal folds. At the posterior aspect of the larynx are found the aryepiglottic, transverse arytenoid, oblique arytenoid, and posterior cricoarytenoid muscles. At the superficial lateral aspect of the larynx are found the cricothyroid muscles. At the deep lateral aspect of the larynx are found the thyroepiglottic, thyroarytenoid, and lateral cricoarytenoid muscles.

Note that most of the muscles of the larynx act to adduct ("close") the true vocal folds. The posterior cricoarytenoid is unique in that it acts to abduct ("open") the true vocal folds. The student should appreciate these muscles from a posterior, lateral, and superior vantage point.

The cricothyroid muscle should be studied in more detail because of some unique characteristics. The cricothyroid muscle originates from the cricoid ring and inserts onto the inferior border of the thyroid cartilage. It acts to draw the thyroid cartilage forward and lengthen the vocal ligaments. It is efferently innervated by the external branch of the superior laryngeal nerve (a branch itself of the vagus nerve).

The cricothyroid muscle is the only intrinsic muscle of the larynx which is supplied by the superior laryngeal nerve. Recall that the superior laryngeal nerve is primarily supplying afferent innervation to the laryngeal mucosa superior to the vocal folds via its internal branch.

All other intrinsic muscles of the larynx are innervated by the recurrent laryngeal nerve (which is also a branch of the vagus nerve) after it has become the inferior laryngeal nerve within the larynx. The inferior laryngeal nerve efferently serves all the other intrinsic muscles of the larynx as well as afferently serving the laryngeal mucosa inferior to the vocal folds.

Damage to the external branch of the superior laryngeal nerve or to the cricothyroid muscle will result in the inability to obtain high pitch during speech. In other words, the opera singer will be unable to hit the high notes and speech becomes monotonous.

Laryngeal Innervation

The recurrent laryngeal nerve supplies sensory (afferent) innervation to the mucosa below the vocal folds as well as motor (efferent) innervation to all of the intrinsic musculature of the larynx except the cricothyroid, which is efferently served by the external branch of the superior laryngeal nerve. Damage to the recurrent laryngeal nerve results in changes to the voice (such as hoarseness), airway problems, and swallowing difficulties.

The superior laryngeal nerve (a branch of the vagus nerve) supplies afferent innervation to the mucosa above the vocal folds as well as motor innervation to the cricothyroid muscle.

Laryngeal Vasculature

The larynx is supplied (vascularly) by the superior and inferior laryngeal arteries.

The superior laryngeal artery is a branch of the superior thyroid artery and accompanies the internal branch of the superior laryngeal nerve through the thyrohyoid membrane superior to the vocal folds.

The inferior laryngeal artery is a branch of the inferior thyroid artery and accompanies the recurrent laryngeal nerve into the laryngeal space inferior to the vocal folds.

Sources Cited:

1-7. Gest, et al. Anatomy Tables (electronic MedCharts). Ann Arbor, MI. 2000

Laboratory Approach

☐1. Examine the styloid musculature, its unique innervation, and its relationship to surrounding pharyngeal structures.

☐2. Describe the neurovasculature of the pharynx including the ascending pharyngeal and palatine arteries, the pharyngeal plexus of nerves, and the pharyngeal plexus of veins.

☐3. Examine the musculature of the soft palate. Describe its relationship to the pharynx as well as the auditory tube.

☐4. Examine the musculature of the pharyngeal wall including the superior, middle, and inferior constrictors. Describe their attachments anteriorly and posteriorly, fiber orientation, and how they attach to the skull base.

☐5. Examine the anatomy of the larynx including its muscular, skeletal, and mucosal components.

☐6. Examine the specific muscles of the larynx (intrinsic and extrinsic) and their actions in opening/closure of the aditus and their actions in vocal fold movement in speech.

☐7. Examine the surface features of the larynx and laryngopharynx.

Pharyngeal Wall

    Muscles of the pharynx
      Stylohyoid (innervated by CN VII) and underlying ligament
      Styloglossus (innervated by CN XII)
      Stylopharyngeus (innervated by CN IX)
      Levator veli palatini
      Tensor veli palatini
         dilator tubae
      Superior pharyngeal constrictor
         associated fasciae
            pharyngobasilar
            buccopharyngeal
         muscular portions
            pterygopharyngeus
            buccopharyngeus
            mylopharyngeus
            glossopharyngeus
      Middle pharyngeal constrictor
      Inferior pharyngeal constrictor
         cricopharyngeus

    Auditory tube (eustachian tube, pharyngotympanic tube)
      Cartilaginous portion
         medial & lateral cartilaginous laminae
      Membranous portion

    Neurovascular structures of the pharynx
      Glossopharyngeal n. (CN IX)
      Vagus n. (CN X)
         Pharyngeal neural plexus
      Ascending pharyngeal a. (branch of external carotid a.)
      Ascending palatine a. (branch of facial a.)
      Pharyngeal venous plexus

Larynx

Membranes & ligaments of the upper airway
    Thyrohyoid membrane
    Quadrangular membrane
    Conus elasticus
    Elastic lamina of the trachea
    Cricothyroid ligament

Pharyngeal features of the larynx
    Laryngopharynx
    Laryngeal aditus
    Interarytenoid notch
    Aryepiglottic fold
    Piriform recess

Internal features of the larynx
    Epiglottis
    Vestibule
    Vestibular fold (false vocal fold)
        rima vestibuli
    Ventricle
    Vocal fold (true vocal fold)
        glottis
        rima glottidis
    Infraglottic cavity

Muscles
    Cricothyroid
    Posterior cricoarytenoideus
    Arytenoideus (oblique and transverse fibers)
    Aryepiglotticus
    Lateral cricoarytenoideus
    Thyroepiglotticus
    Thyroarytenoideus
        Vocalis (and underlying vocal ligament)

Vagus n. (CN X)
    Superior laryngeal n.
        external branch
        internal branch
    Recurrent laryngeal n.
        inferior laryngeal n.

Vasculature
  Superior laryngeal a. (from superior thyroid a.)
  Inferior laryngeal a. (from inferior thyroid a.)

Orbit

Introduction

This chapter will study the orbit and its contents, as well as the cavernous sinus.

The orbit is the cone shaped space in the midface region which contains the globe (a.k.a. "eye"), its neurovascular supply, the extraocular muscles controlling the globe's movements, and autonomically controlled glands and smooth muscles.

The retina of the globe is afferently innervated by the optic nerve (CN II), while the extraocular muscles which control the globe's movements are efferently served by the oculomotor, trochlear, and abducens nerves (CN III, IV, and VI, respectively).

Autonomic control to the globe is via cranial nerve III, while general afferents to the globe are via cranial nerve V-1 (the ophthalmic division).

Bony Orbit

The orbit is composed of seven primary bones.

Its "rim" is its most superficial region, and creates the circular entrance into the orbital space from an external approach. This rim is composed of contributions from the frontal, zygomatic, and maxillary bones.

The deepest portion of the orbit (a.k.a. its "apex") is composed from contributions from the sphenoid, ethmoid, lacrimal, and palatine bones.

The roof of the orbit is directly inferior to the anterior cranial fossa, while the floor of the orbit is directly superior to the maxillary sinus.

A line through the long axis of the orbit would not run directly anterior to posterior. Instead, it would be an obliquely oriented line passing from anterior to posterior and lateral to medial. In other words, lines passing through the long axis of each orbit would meet posterior to the orbital spaces since they are not parallel to each other.

The optic nerve arrives in the orbital space through the optic canal which is at the apex of the orbit. The oculomotor nerve, trochlear nerve, abducens nerve, and ophthalmic division of the trigeminal nerve arrive in the orbital space through the superior orbital fissure.

The lacrimal bones and maxillary bones create a space which holds the lacrimal sac at the medial aspect of the orbit. This lacrimal sac is the structure which the tears, which originate from the lacrimal gland, will drain into. This sac will be discussed in further detail later in this chapter, but you should appreciate the bony space in which it sits at this point. The lacrimal gland will also be discussed in further detail, and is found at the superolateral aspect of the orbital space immediately posterior to the orbital rim.

The ophthalmic artery (a branch of the internal carotid artery) and optic nerve travel into the orbital space via the optic canal.

Cranial nerves III, IV, V-1, and VI travel into the orbital space via the superior orbital fissure.

Ophthalmic veins travel through the orbit via the superior and inferior orbital fissures.

Note the thinness of both the orbital roof (inferior to the anterior cranial fossa) and the orbital floor (superior to the maxillary sinus space).

Eye Within the Orbit

The bulbus oculi (a.k.a. the "globe" or "eye") lies at the anterior aspect of the orbital space. The eyelids are immediately anterior to the globe, and are anchored to the orbital rim via the orbital septum.

The eyelids serve to keep the globe moistened and to protect it from injury and trauma. From superficial to deep, the eyelids are composed of skin, orbicularis oculi musculature, tarsal plates, and an internal conjunctival lining.

The tarsal plates give the eyelids their "bulk", and are composed of connective tissue. The orbital septum is a thin layer of periosteum which extends into the tarsal plates from the bony rim of the orbit. It anchors the eyelids to the orbital rim.

The conjunctiva is a thin layer of membranous tissue which covers the internal aspect of the eyelids (palpebral portion) and the anterior external aspect of the globe (bulbar portion). Since the conjunctiva only covers the anterior surface of the globe, it ends in a superior and inferior "blind alley" called the conjunctival fornix. The region in between these fornices is known as the conjunctival sac.

The area posterior to the globe is filled with extraocular muscles and orbital fat. This fat serves to protect the globe, as does the bulbar fascia on the posterior aspect of the globe.

The periorbital fat is loosely arranged within a connective tissue matrix. This is important clinically in cases of injury or trauma as fluid can accumulate in this space.

External Features of the Eye

The area near the nasal bridge where the superior and inferior eyelids meet is called the medial canthus. The area where the superior and inferior eyelids meet laterally is called the lateral canthus. The space between the superior and inferior eyelids is called the palpebral fissure. It is this fissure which you open and close as you "blink".

The white of the globe is called the sclera. The opening at the anterior aspect of the globe which allows light into the globe is called the pupil. The set of colored muscular fibers (which are both radial and circular) around the pupil is called the iris. The transparent layer of tissue overlying the pupil and iris is the cornea.

At the medial canthus is found the lacrimal caruncle within the lacrimal lake. This small protuberance contains modified sebaceous glandular tissue. The plica semilunaris is immediately lateral to the caruncle.

Superficial Dissection of the Orbit

Directly deep to the skin of the orbital rim and eyelids are found the orbicularis oculi muscles. These muscles are muscles of facial expression, and are therefore efferently served by the facial nerve (temporal and zygomatic branches). They act to close the eyelids. They can be divided into an orbital part (overlying orbital bone) and a palpebral part (overlying the tarsal plates of the eyelids).

The angles of the eyelids (those regions at the medial and lateral canthi) are anchored to the underlying orbital rim via medial and lateral palpebral ligaments.

The orbicularis oculi muscles attach to both the orbital rim and the palpebral ligaments. The palpebral portions of the muscles are responsible for "normal" blinking actions of the eyelids while the orbital portions are responsible for "forced" blinking.

It is important to note that the lacrimal sac lies deep to the medial palpebral ligament at the medial aspect of the orbit. There are orbicularis oculi fibers anterior and posterior to the lacrimal sac.

Notice, like the orbicularis oculi, how the tarsal plates are anchored to orbital bone via the medial and lateral palpebral ligaments. These ligaments anchor the plates medially and laterally.

With the removal of the skin and musculature, the orbital septum can be readily visualized. This extension of the orbital periosteum anchors the tarsal plates superiorly and inferiorly.

Deep to the orbital septum in the superolateral aspect of the orbit is the lacrimal gland.

The upper eyelid is opened via the levator palpebrae superioris muscle which originates at the orbital apex superior to the optic canal. It inserts into the musculature and tarsal plate of the upper eyelid. It is efferently served by the oculomotor nerve. Its distal-most fibers are actually smooth muscle (sometimes called the "superior tarsal muscle fibers") which are sympathetically innervated. Make special note that the levator palpebrae superioris fibers actually pass through the orbital septum to attach into the superior aspect of the tarsal plate.

There are glands deep to the tarsal plates, and there are also glands at the roots of the eyelashes. These are sebaceous glands which secret an oily substance serving the region. Infections in the lash follicles and tarsal glands are called styes and chalazions (respectively). The lacrimal sac resides deep to the medial palpebral ligament. It is important to recall that fibers of the orbicularis oculi lie both anterior and posterior to the lacrimal sac. The corresponding lacrimal gland is located in the superolateral aspect of the orbit.

Lacrimation

There are small openings on the upper and lower eyelids called puncta. These puncta are surrounded by a protuberant papillae and are at the medial canthus. They are essentially the external openings of small tubes called lacrimal canaliculi which connect the conjunctival sac to the lacrimal sac.

Tears are produced by the lacrimal gland in the superolateral aspect of the orbit. These tears wash from superior to inferior and from lateral to medial across the globe within the conjunctival sac. They are then drawn into the puncta and travel through the canaliculi until they reach the lacrimal sac. Once in the lacrimal sac, the tears can travel inferiorly through the nasolacrimal duct where they ultimately drain into the inferior nasal meatus (which will be studied in a subsequent chapter) in the nasal cavity.

The lacrimal gland is innervated (parasympathetically) by the facial nerve (with postganglionic fibers arising from the pterygopalatine ganglia in the pterygopalatine fossa). The course of this innervation will be further studied later in this chapter.

The lacrimal sac draws in tears via vacuum action. This action is initiated as the eyelids are blinked. Contraction of the orbicularis oculi fibers posterior the lacrimal sac cause the sac to enlarge between the orbicularis oculi fibers and the medial palpebral ligament. This enlargement creates a vacuum within the lacrimal sac and draws tears from the conjunctival sac through the puncta and canaliculi into the lacrimal sac. Therefore, closure of the eyelids assists in drawing tears into the lacrimal sac.

Lacrimal Innervation: Preganglionic parasympathetic fibers from the facial nerve (via the greater petrosal nerve) arrive at the posterior wall of the pterygopalatine ganglion after having exited the skull via the foramen lacerum. They join with postganglionic sympathetic fibers (via the deep petrosal nerve) to become the nerve of the pterygoid canal. The nerve of the pterygoid canal arrives at the pterygopalatine ganglion through the posterior wall of the pterygopalatine fossa. There, the sympathetic fibers pass through (having already synapsed in the superior cervical ganglion), and the parasympathetic fibers synapse with their postganglionic counterparts. Both sets of postganglionic autonomic fibers then "hitch a ride" with the maxillary division of the trigeminal nerve (V2) as it travels through the inferior orbital floor and maxillary sinus roof. They then jump onto the zygomatic nerve and travel to the lacrimal gland in the orbit.

NOTE: Textbooks typically show autonomic fibers jumping off from the zygomatic nerve and onto the lacrimal nerve (a branch of V1 within the orbit) before reaching the lacrimal gland. While this can occur, the zygomatic nerve can also deliver autonomic fibers directly to the lacrimal gland.

Orbital Innervation

The optic canal allows for the passage of the optic nerve into the orbital space. It should be noted that the internal carotid canal is immediately posterior to the optic canal.

The superior orbital fissure is found inferolateral to the optic canal. It allows for the passage of the oculomotor nerve, the trochlear nerve, branches of V1, and the abducens nerve. Ophthalmic veins also pass through this fissure.

Take time to review all of the various openings on the internal and external aspect of the skull and know what structures traverse the openings.

Notice the relationship between the pituitary gland, the optic nerve, and the internal carotid artery. The artery resides immediately posterior to the optic nerve, and it lies immediately lateral to the pituitary gland.

The cavernous sinus also lies posterior and lateral to the pituitary gland. Cranial nerves III, IV, V1, V2, and VI lie within the cavernous sinus. The internal carotid artery also lies within the cavernous sinus.

The optic nerve takes back afferent information from the globe to the central nervous system and is the primary nerve involved in sight. It communicates directly with the retina which is found along the posterior surface of the inner eye.

The oculomotor, trochlear, and abducens nerves efferently innervate extraocular muscles which act to move the globe within the orbital space. The mnemonic "$SO_4LR_6AO_3$" allows one to readily remember that the superior oblique muscle is innervated by the trochlear nerve (CN IV), the lateral rectus muscle is innervated by the abducens nerve (CN VI), and that all the other extraocular muscles are innervated by the oculomotor nerve (CN III).

Immediately superior to the levator palpebrae superioris can be found the frontal nerve. This nerve is a branch of V-1 and afferently serves the skin of the forehead and the upper eyelid after terminating into the supraorbital and supratrochlear nerves (which ultimately leave the orbital space to reach cutaneous tissues).

Also immediately superior to the levator palpebrae superioris is the lacrimal nerve. The lacrimal nerve, like the frontal nerve, is a branch of V-1 and is located lateral to the frontal nerve in the same plane. It is immediately superior to the lateral rectus muscle. This nerve afferently serves the conjunctiva and also carries postganglionic parasympathetic fibers from the pterygopalatine ganglion. The postganglionic fibers which travel with the lacrimal nerve hitch a ride onto it after having hitched a ride with the zygomatic branch of V-2 following their exit from the pterygopalatine ganglion.

More medially located, but within the same general plane, one can find the trochlear nerve (CN IV) on its way to efferently innervate the superior oblique muscle.

The nasociliary nerve resides deep within the orbit. This is another branch of V-1, but it enters the orbital space within the common tendinous ring (unlike the frontal and lacrimal nerves which enter external to the ring). It is found deep to the superior rectus muscle and will be better visualized in subsequent slides. It is mentioned here because it is one of the three major branches of V-1 within the orbit. The three major branches of V-1 are the frontal, lacrimal, and nasociliary nerves.

General afferent sensation to the orbit and its contents arises from the ophthalmic division of the trigeminal nerve (primarily) and the maxillary division of the trigeminal nerve (in a minor way through the orbital floor).

Parasympathetic supply to the orbit is supplied by the oculomotor nerve (via the ciliary ganglion) and the facial nerve (via the pterygopalatine ganglion). Sympathetic supply is supplied by the postganglionic sympathetics from the superior cervical ganglion.

Orbital Vasculature

Entering into the orbital space with the optic nerve (deep to the superior rectus muscle) is the ophthalmic artery. This artery is the first branch of the internal carotid artery and branches off from the internal carotid within the cranial vault.

The ophthalmic artery has many named branches within the orbit.

One of the most important branches of the ophthalmic artery is the central artery of the retina. This artery dives into the substance of the optic nerve and supplies the posterointernal surface of the globe (the retina). This artery is unique in that is the only artery in the human body which is directly visible to the clinician (via an ophthalmoscope and fundoscopic examination). The central artery of the retina is the sole blood supply to the retina and has no significant collateral circulation. Damage to it (or blockage of its flow) leads to retinal damage (blindness).

Other important branches include the anterior and posterior ethmoidal arteries which travel to the lateral wall of the nasal cavity through ethmoid bone and will be studied in detail in a later chapter.

The orbit also contains many venous structures. Some of these structures are serving the globe and orbit. Others are merely passing through the orbital space and anastomose with orbital veins.

The inferior and superior ophthalmic veins pass through the orbit and connect veins of the midface (such as the angular and pterygoid plexus veins) with the cavernous sinus. It is through these venous channels that pathology can spread from the superficial face to the internal aspect of the skull and cavernous sinus space.

Study specifically the location of the cavernous sinus as well as its communications with the midface (via ophthalmic and pterygoid veins) and also with deeper venous sinus spaces (via petrosal sinus connections). The cavernous sinus partially encircles the pituitary gland in the middle cranial fossa.

Various cranial nerves exit the cranial vault by passing through the cavernous sinus space. These nerves include CN III, IV, V-1 and V-2, as well as VI.

The internal carotid artery also passes through the cavernous sinus space.

It is important to note that most structures passing through the sinus pass through along its lateral walls. The internal carotid artery and abducens nerve, however, pass through the center of the cavernous sinus.

If any infection sets up shop in the cavernous sinus space (from an infected facial laceration, for example), the blood in the sinus may clot (thrombose) and an abscess may form. This is clinically significant because the internal carotid artery may be compromised (leading to a hemorrhagic stroke) if the infection erodes through its walls. The abducens nerve may also be compromised leading to the inability to abduct the eye on the affected side (given the role of CN VI in efferently serving the lateral rectus muscle). Structures along the lateral wall of the cavernous sinus space are largely unaffected in such circumstances.

Infections of the cavernous sinus can be treated with antibiotics, but abscesses sometimes can be difficult to eradicate without physical evacuation of the infection.

Orbital Musculature

The most superficial muscle encountered is the levator palpebrae superioris. Recall that it is an elevator of the upper eyelid and is efferently innervated by the oculomotor nerve (superior division). Immediately deep to the levator palpebrae superioris is the superior rectus muscle. This muscle is also efferently innervated by the superior division of the oculomotor nerve. It originates from a common tendinous ring at the apex of the orbit and inserts into the superior surface of the globe. It elevates and adducts the globe.

Medially, the superior oblique muscle may be seen. The superior oblique originates from the common tendinous ring at the apex of the orbit and inserts into the superoposterior surface of the globe. It depresses and abducts the globe and is efferently innervated by the trochlear nerve. This muscle is unique in that it passes through a fibrocartilaginous pulley called the trochlea at the antero-medial aspect of the orbit. Contraction of the muscle through the trochlea redirects force vectors in such a way as to move the eye "down and out".

Additionally, the medial rectus muscle can be seen inferior to the superior oblique muscle on the medial aspect of the orbit. The medial rectus originates from the common tendinous ring at the apex of the orbit and inserts into the medial surface of the globe. It adducts the globe and is efferently innervated by the inferior division of the oculomotor nerve.

Laterally, the lateral rectus muscle can be seen. The lateral rectus originates from the common tendinous ring at the apex of the orbit and inserts onto the lateral aspect of the globe. It acts to abduct the globe and is efferently innervated by the abducens nerve.

The inferior rectus muscle originates at the common tendinous ring at the apex of the orbit and inserts onto the inferior surface of the globe. It acts to depress the globe and is efferently innervated by the inferior division of the oculomotor nerve.

The inferior oblique muscle originates from the floor of the orbit and inserts onto the inferior surface of the globe. It acts to elevate and abduct the globe (or to turn the eye "up and out"). It is efferently innervated by the inferior division of the oculomotor nerve.

Specifically note the fiber orientation of the superior and inferior oblique muscles. Because of their insertion points onto the globe they serve to move the eye "down and out" (superior oblique) and "up and out" (inferior oblique). Pay close attention to the movements afforded by the obliques. They may seem counterintuitive at first, but arise given the attachment points of the musculature to the globe.

All of the extraocular muscles arise from the common tendinous ring at the apex of the orbit with the exception of the inferior oblique (which arises from the orbital floor). The common tendinous ring divides the superior orbital fissure into two parts. One part is within the ring, and the other is external to it. The optic canal is entirely within the common tendinous ring. The inferior orbital fissure is entirely outside (external to) the common tendinous ring. Note specifically that the optic nerve, oculomotor nerve, and abducens nerve pass through the superior orbital fissure within the ring. A branch of V-1 (the nasociliary nerve) also passes through the superior orbital fissure within the ring. The trochlear nerve and other branches of V-1 (the lacrimal and frontal nerves) enter the orbit through the superior orbital fissure, but do so external to the ring.

Orbital Autonomics

The oculomotor nerve serves to supply the globe with parasympathetic innervation. The ciliary muscles (attaching to the optic lens) and the sphincter pupillae muscles (circular muscle fibers in the iris) are innervated by parasympathetic fibers from the oculomotor nerve. Preganglionic parasympathetic fibers from the oculomotor nerve travel to the ciliary ganglion, and following synapse in the ciliary ganglion, postganglionic parasympathetics pass to the globe via short ciliary nerves. These short ciliary nerves also carry postganglionic sympathetic fibers (serving the radial dilator fibers in the iris) as well as general afferents from the nasociliary nerve.

Long ciliary nerves contain both general afferents to the globe (from the nasociliary nerve) as well as postganglionic sympathetic fibers from the superior cervical ganglion. The long ciliary nerves, however, do not carry parasympathetic fibers.

The iris contains circular fibers (the sphincter pupillae muscles) which are parasympathetically innervated (and which constrict the pupillary opening) and radial fibers (the dilator pupillae muscles) which are sympathetically innervated (and which dilate or open the pupillary opening).

The ciliary muscles are also parasympathetically innervated. These muscles attach to the optic lens and serve to relax the suspensory ligaments of the lens when contracted. Contraction actually relaxes the suspensory ligaments allowing for the lens to thicken and accommodate (for "up close" or "near vision").

Laboratory Approach

☐1. Examine the seven extraocular muscles and their attachments and neurovascular supply.

☐2. Examine the smooth musculature of the orbit and eye and describe their autonomic innervation and functional roles.

☐3. Examine the general innervation to the orbit and eye. Specifically examine and trace CN III, IV, VI, V2, and VI with all relevant branches.

☐4. Examine the vascular supply to the orbit and eye. Specifically examine the ophthalmic artery and its branches.

☐5. Examine the lacrimal apparatus of the orbit and be able to describe lacrimation and the flow of tears into the inferior nasal meatus.

☐6. Examine the osteology of the orbit and describe the regional location of the orbit in relation to the nasal cavity, paranasal sinuses, and cranial fossae.

☐7. Examine the cavernous sinus and describe where specific structures within the sinus are located.

External features of the eye
    Medial & lateral canthus
    Superior & inferior conjunctival fornices
    Bulbar & palpebral conjunctiva
    Cornea
        Sclera
        Pupil
        Iris

Lacrimal apparatus
    Lacrimal gland
    Lacrimal canaliculi
    Lacrimal papillae
        Lacrimal puncta
    Lacrimal caruncle
    Lacrimal sac
    Nasolacrimal duct

Nerves
    Optic n. (CN II)
    Oculomotor n. (CN III)
        superior division
        inferior division
            communicating branches to the ciliary ganglion
    Ciliary ganglion
        short ciliary nn.
    Trochlear n. (CN IV)
    Ophthalmic division (V1) of the trigeminal n.
        lacrimal n.
            communicating branches from zygomatic n. (V2)
        frontal n.
            supratrochlear n.
            supraorbital (medial and lateral branches) n.
        nasociliary n.
            long ciliary nn.
            anterior & posterior ethmoidal nn.
            external nasal n.
            infratrochlear n.
    Maxillary division (V2) of the trigeminal n.
    Abducens n. (CN VI)

Vessels
    Ophthalmic veins (superior & inferior)
    Ophthalmic a.
        central artery of the retina
        anterior & posterior ethmoidal aa.

Muscles
    Extraocular
        levator palpebrae superioris
            superior tarsal (smooth muscle)
        rectus mm.
            superior, inferior, medial and lateral
        superior oblique (& trochlea)
        inferior oblique
        orbicularis oculi (NOTE: this is NOT one of the extraoculars but is
                regional and important)
   Intraocular (smooth muscle)
       dilator pupillae (sympathetic)
       sphincter pupillae (parasympathetic)
         ciliary (parasympathetic)

Miscellaneous
    Ciliary apparatus
    Tarsal plate
    Anulus tendineus
    Orbital septum
    Periorbita (orbital periosteum)
    Cavernous sinus
        Internal carotid a.
        CN III, IV, V1, V2, VI

ETHMOID BONE
Perpendicular plate
Cribriform plate
Ethmoidal hiatus
Crista galli
Orbital lamina
Middle nasal concha
Anterior and posterior ethmoidal foramina
Ethmoidal bulla
Superior nasal concha

LACRIMAL BONE
Lacrimal sulcus
Posterior lacrimal crest

Nasal Cavity and the Oral Cavity

Introduction

This chapter will study the oral and nasal cavities and their contents.

Recall that the pharyngeal spaces all lie posterior to the various cavities (oral cavity, nasal cavity, and laryngeal cavity/larynx). The laryngeal cavity has already been studied in a previous chapter. The oral and nasal cavities will be studied in more detail in this chapter.

The nasal cavity lies entirely superior to the hard palate. It also lies inferomedial to the orbit. It is directly inferior to the anterior cranial fossa. It is divided into two distinct sub-cavities (a right and a left) via the nasal septum.

The nasal septum is a bony and cartilaginous structure passing between the left and right nasal cavities. The choanae mark the entrance between the nasal cavity and the nasopharynx. Recall that the auditory tube opens into the nasopharynx immediately posterior to the nasal cavity and superior to the soft palate.

As an introduction, it should be noted that the neurovasculature of the nasal cavity is relatively straight-forward. The general afferent innervation of the nasal cavity is supplied by V-1 and V-2 fibers. The blood supply to the region is supplied by branches of the facial, maxillary, and ophthalmic arteries.

The nasal cavity also contains the nerves responsible for olfaction ("smell"). At the roof of the nasal cavity can be found branches of the olfactory nerve (CN I) supplying the olfactory epithelium.

There are various air spaces called parasagittal sinuses (a.k.a. "paranasal sinuses") in the regions around the nasal cavity. These should be examined as they are approached regionally.

The oral cavity lies inferior to the hard palate and nasal cavities. The entrance between the oral cavity and the oropharynx is the called the fauces.

The oral cavity is served by V-2 and V-3 afferent nerve fibers and is served arterially by branches of the facial, lingual, and palatine arteries.

Nasal Cavity

The region superior to the hard palate and anterior to the vibrating line (the junction between the hard and soft palates) is the nasal cavity. That region posterior to the vibrating line and superior to the soft palate is the nasopharynx.

Pharyngeal tonsil tissue is found at the posterosuperior aspect of the nasopharynx, while the palatine tonsil tissue is found within the oropharynx. Recall that the palatine tonsils are located between the palatoglossal and palatopharyngeal folds. These folds are created by the oral mucosa which overlies the palatoglossus and palatopharyngeus muscles. These two muscles both originate from the palatine aponeurosis. One inserts into the tongue (palatoglossus) while the other inserts into the posterior wall of the pharynx (palatopharyngeus). Both muscles elevate that which they insert into, and both are efferently served by the vagus nerve (CN X). (1, Muscles of the Head and Neck - Palatoglossus and Palatopharyngeus)

The lateral nasal wall contains the superior, middle, and inferior concha. These mucosa covered bony protuberances serve to disrupt the flow of air through the nasal cavity allowing it to be moisturized and warmed before reaching the lower airway. They also give inhaled air more time to pass over the olfactory mucosa at the superior aspect of the nasal cavity (ensuring better olfaction).

The spaces immediately inferior to each concha are called meatuses. There are, therefore, superior, middle, and inferior nasal meatuses.

The superior and middle nasal concha arise from ethmoid bone. The inferior nasal concha is its own bone (and does not arise from another named bone).

The septum is formed from bone (ethmoid, maxillary, palatine, and vomer bones) as well as cartilage (at its anterior region). Clinically, this cartilage is important because it can be harvested for use in reconstructive surgery ("plastic surgery").

Nasal Vasculature

There is an intricate network of nerves and blood vessels supplying the nasal cavity.

Know now that the nasal cavity is highly innervated and highly vascularized. Most of the distal branches of the nerves and arteries which supply the nasal cavity will not be visible on any cadaveric specimen due to embalming procedures, post-mortem swelling, and the small caliber of the branches.

The sphenopalatine foramen can be found at the posterosuperior aspect of the nasal cavity allowing passage of the sphenopalatine artery. The sphenopalatine artery supplies the posterior and inferior aspect of the nasal septum and the lateral nasal wall. The branch of the sphenopalatine artery which supplies the posteroinferior nasal septum is the posterior septal nasal branch. The branch of the sphenopalatine artery which supplies the posteroinferior lateral nasal wall is the posterior lateral nasal branch(es).

Notice that both the anterosuperior septum and anterosuperior lateral nasal walls are supplied by the anterior and posterior ethmoidal arteries (which originated in the orbit from the ophthalmic artery).

Thus, the ophthalmic artery supplies the anterosuperior nasal cavity while the maxillary artery (via the sphenopalatine artery) supplies the posteroinferior nasal cavity.

Deep (lateral) to the posterior lateral nasal wall can be found the pterygopalatine fossa. A palatine canal leaves this fossa bed and travels to the posterior aspect of the hard palate (bilaterally). It is through this canal which the descending palatine artery travels (after branching from the maxillary artery in the pterygopalatine fossa space). The descending palatine artery then splits into the greater (anterior) and lesser (posterior) palatine arteries.

These arteries serve the palate.

The greater palatine artery anastomoses with nasal branches of the sphenopalatine artery at the anterior portion of the palate.

Kiesselbach's plexus is a set of tiny blood vessels found at the anterior septal region which is highly vascularized and the most common site of epistaxis (nosebleeds). It is an anastomotic region connecting branches of the facial artery, the ethmoidal arteries, and the sphenopalatine artery.

The palatine blood vessels travel with palatine nerves (greater and lesser palatine nerves originally from V-2 in the pterygopalatine fossa) through the palatine canal.

Nasal Innervation

At the posterior aspect of the lateral nasal wall, the pterygopalatine fossa can be found. The pterygopalatine ganglion can be found within the fossa space. V-2 also passes through this space and the ganglion is attached and connected to V-2.

Branches from V-2 (which may pass through the ganglion given its proximity) enter the nasal cavity through the sphenopalatine foramen and supply the posteroinferior nasal cavity.

The branch of V-2 which serves the posteroinferior nasal septum is the nasopalatine nerve. Branches of V-2 also serve the lateral nasal wall and arise from more distal V-2 branches (such as the palatine nerves). The anterior ethmoidal nerve (from the nasociliary nerve in the orbit) serves the anterosuperior nasal septum and lateral nasal wall. Thus V-1 (anterosuperiorly) and V-2 (poster-inferiorly) afferently serve the nasal cavity.

The olfactory nerve supplies the nasal cavity with olfaction at the nasal cavity roof.

Note that branches of V-2 from the pterygopalatine fossa travel inferiorly within the palatine canal to reach the posterior portion of the hard palate where they exit (with the previously studied palatine arteries) via the greater and lesser palatine foramina. The greater palatine nerve then serves the hard palate anteriorly while the lesser palatine nerve travels posteriorly to serve the soft palate.

Paranasal Sinuses

Paranasal spaces are lined with mucosa and are cavitations within the bones of the midface region (frontal, ethmoid, maxillary, and sphenoid bones). They are named "paranasal" because they communicate with the nasal cavity.

These sinuses are largely absent in the neonate and develop as maturation and development progresses.

Important sinuses are the frontal sinuses, the sphenoidal sinuses, the maxillary sinuses, and the ethmoidal air cells.

Beneath the superior, middle, and inferior nasal conchae are the superior, middle, and inferior meatuses. Within these meatuses are openings into the paranasal sinuses and the lacrimal sac.

The nasolacrimal duct (originating from the lacrimal sac) empties into the inferior nasal meatus. This is the only opening in the inferior nasal meatus.

The middle nasal meatus has four sets of openings within itself. One of these openings is the ostium of the maxillary sinus. This opening is at the superior aspect of the maxillary sinus. Another opening within the middle nasal meatus is the ostium of the nasofrontal duct at the anterosuperior portion of the semilunar hiatus. This opening leads into the frontal sinus. There are also two sets of openings within the middle meatus which allow passage into the anterior and middle ethmoidal air cells. The bulla ethmoidalis and the hiatus semilunaris (inferior to the bulla ethmoidalis) are also found within the middle meatus. The bulla ethmoidalis leads anteriorly to the ethmoidal infundibulum.

The superior nasal meatus contains a set of openings which allow passage into the posterior ethmoidal air cells.

The ostium of the sphenoid sinus is found at the superoposterior aspect of the nasal cavity and allows passage into the sphenoid sinus space.

The mucosal linings of the paranasal sinuses secrete a mucus necessary to keep the mucosa and nasal cavity moist. This mucus is removed from the paranasal sinus spaces via ciliary action. Interestingly, the only sinus which has dependent drainage is the frontal sinus (and uses gravity with ciliary action to empty its contents). All other sinuses rely on ciliary action alone. (2, p. 125)

Oral Cavity

The opening into the oropharynx from the oral cavity is called the fauces.

At the fauces lie the palatoglossal and palatopharyngeal folds. The palatoglossus and palatopharyngeus muscles are covered in oral mucosa creating these folds. Note that the palatine tonsil tissue nestles between the palatopharyngeal and palatoglossal folds within the oropharynx. This space is called the palatine tonsil bed.

Within the palatine tonsil bed (within the oropharynx) can be seen tonsillar artery branches of the facial artery. The palatine tonsils are supplied by branches from the ascending pharyngeal artery, the facial artery (tonsillar and palatal branches), and the lingual artery. Notice also that the glossopharyngeal nerve (CN IX) passes deep to the palatine tonsil bed. The glossopharyngeal nerve is serving the region afferently. Given the rich vascular supply to the palatine tonsillar bed and the underlying glossopharyngeal nerve, surgical procedures (such as palatine tonsil resection) in the region are relatively risky.

The hard and soft palates lie superoanterior to the fauces in the oral cavity. The greater and lesser palatine arteries serve the hard and soft palates, respectively. These arteries mirror the palatine nerves in many ways.

The uvula hangs down at the posterior aspect of the soft palate and is composed of soft palatal tissue. It acts as a valve closing the opening into the nasopharynx from the oropharynx upon swallowing.

Infratemporal Fossa and Pterygopalatine Fossa

The infratemporal fossa has been studied in detail in other chapters and should be reviewed here. It is important in this context because it contains a special opening along its deep (medial) wall. This opening is the pterygomaxillary fissure (between the lateral pterygoid plate and the posterior maxillary border). It is through this fissure that branches of the maxillary artery begin their journey to the nasal cavity.

The pterygomaxillary fissure is essentially the "doorway" to the pterygopalatine fossa from a lateral approach. Recall that this fossa space is where V-2 and the pterygopalatine ganglia can also be found. The medial wall of the pterygopalatine fossa houses the sphenopalatine foramen which is itself a "doorway" into the lateral aspect of the nasal cavity.

The sphenopalatine artery (from the maxillary artery) passes through the pterygomaxillary fissure, through the pterygopalatine fossa, and ultimately through the sphenopalatine foramen on its way to the nasal cavity.

Branches of V-2 gain access to the nasal cavity after passing through the pterygopalatine fossa and the sphenopalatine foramen. The do not, however, pass through the pterygomaxillary fissure on their journey. Instead, they enter the pterygopalatine fossa through its posterior wall (which is where the foramen rotundum ends) before diving medially through the sphenopalatine foramen to enter the nasal cavity.

Midface Arterial Supply: Maxillary Artery

The maxillary artery can be seen in the infratemporal fossa. Recall that 50% of the time it lies lateral to the lateral pterygoid muscle, and 50% of the time it lies deep to the lateral pterygoid muscle.

The distal portion of the maxillary artery travels anteriorly until it reaches the pterygomaxillary fissure where it passes through the fissure opening to gain access to the pterygopalatine fossa as the sphenopalatine artery. The sphenopalatine artery then travels medially (deeply) to exit the pterygopalatine fossa through the sphenopalatine foramen.

The sphenopalatine foramen allows the sphenopalatine artery to reach the nasal cavity. Traveling with the sphenopalatine artery to the nasal cavity (through the sphenopalatine foramen) is the nasopalatine nerve (a branch of V-2 serving the nasal cavity).

Take time to review the other branches of the maxillary artery which were covered in previous chapters. Also recall that the maxillary artery is terminal branch of the external carotid artery (as is the superficial temporal artery).

Sources Cited:

1. Gest, et al. Anatomy Tables (electronic MedCharts). Ann Arbor, MI. 2000

2. Brzezinski, et al. Laboratory and Study Guide for Head and Neck Anatomy: Dissection of the Head and Neck. Ann Arbor, MI. 2013

Laboratory Approach

☐1. Examine the nasal cavity and the nasopharynx identifying surface features of the nasal septum and the lateral nasal wall.

☐2. Examine the paranasal sinuses and the bones that enclose them as well as their relationships to the lateral nasal wall. Identify and describe the openings of the paranasal sinuses into the nasal cavity.

☐3. Examine and describe the neurovascular supply to the nasal cavity.

☐4. Examine the musculature of the soft palate and its neurovascular supply.

☐5. Examine the lingual, pharyngeal, and palatine tonsils and describe the vascular supply to each.

☐6. Examine the hard palate and its neurovascular supply.

☐7. Examine the fauces and muscular folds which mark the separation between the oral cavity and the oropharynx.

Key Regional Structures

Nerves & vessels (by region)

Superior region
Arteries
ophthalmic a.
anterior & posterior ethmoidal
septal branches
lateral nasal branches
Nerves
anterior ethmoidal n. (V1)
external nasal
internal nasal
septal branches
lateral branches
olfactory nn. (CN 1)

Posterior region
Arteries
maxillary a. (third part)
sphenopalatine
posterior septal branches
posterior lateral branches
Nerves
posterior superior nasal (V2)
lateral branches
septal branches (nasopalatine n.)
posterior inferior lateral nasal (V2)

Anterior inferior region
Arteries
facial a.
superior labial
septal and vestibular branches
Nerves
anterior superior alveolar
infraorbital n. (V2)

Nasal septum
Vomer
Ethmoid, perpendicular plate
Septal cartilage

Lateral nasal wall
Sphenoethmoidal recess
ostium, sphenoid sinus
Superior concha (turbinate)
Superior meatus
ostia, posterior ethmoidal air cells
Middle concha (turbinate)

Middle meatus
   bulla ethmoidalis
      ostium, middle ethmoidal air cells
   hiatus semilunaris
   ethmoid infundibulum
     ostia of:
        frontonasal duct
        anterior ethmoidal air cells
        maxillary sinus
Inferior concha (turbinate)
Inferior meatus
     ostium of nasolacrimal duct
Vestibule

Nasopharynx
   Torus tubarius
  Pharyngeal orifice of the auditory tube
  Pharyngeal recess
  Salpingopharyngeal fold
    (salpingopharyngeus m.)

Mucoperiosteum

Hard palate
  Incisive papilla
  Palatine rugae
  Palatine mucous glands (both hard and soft palate)
  Neurovascular supply
    greater palatine a. (maxillary a.) and n. (V2)
    nasopalatine n. (V2)
    septal branch of the sphenopalatine a.

Soft palate (palatal velum)
  Uvula
  Palatal aponeurosis
  Lesser palatine aa. (maxillary a.) and nn. (V2)

Fauces
  Palatoglossal fold (anterior pillar)
  Palatopharyngeal fold (posterior pillar)

Tonsillar fossa (sinus)
  Palatine tonsils
    tonsillar crypts
  Structures of the floor
    superior pharyngeal constrictor m.
    styloglossus m.
    stylohyoid ligament
    middle pharyngeal constrictor m.
    glossopharyngeal n.

Tonsillar arterial branches from:
 descending palatine a. (via the lesser palatine a.)
 ascending palatine a. (facial a.)
 ascending pharyngeal a.
 dorsal lingual a.
 facial a.

Muscles
 Palatoglossus
 Palatopharyngeus
 Musculus uvulae
 Levator veli palatini
 Tensor veli palatini
 Superior and middle pharyngeal constrictor
 Styloglossus

VOMER BONE
Alae
Nasopalatine groove

INFERIOR CONCHA BONE

Trigeminal Nerve and its Branches

Introduction

This chapter will review the three branches of the trigeminal nerve with specific focus on the maxillary division.

The trigeminal nerve is cranial nerve number five. It has both an afferent component and an efferent component.

You should take this time to review all of the cranial nerves and be able to describe whether they are afferent, efferent, or both. You should also be able to describe the functions of each cranial nerve, including any autonomic functions if relevant.

You should also take this time to review the openings and foramina through which each cranial nerve passes. The trigeminal nerve branches pass through the superior orbital fissure (V-1), the foramen rotundum (V-2), and the foramen ovale (V-3).

Trigeminal Nerve Divisions

The ophthalmic division (V-1) is entirely afferent, as is the maxillary division (V-2). The ophthalmic division serves the orbit and cutaneous tissues at and superior to the superior eyelid. The maxillary division serves the midface and its cutaneous tissues (between the inferior eyelid and the upper lip).

The mandibular division (V-3) of the trigeminal nerve is a mixed nerve, and contains both afferent and efferent fibers. Afferently it serves the lower face and its cutaneous tissues (between the lower lip and the base of the mandible). Efferently it serves the muscles of mastication, the tensor muscles (veli palatini of the soft palate and tympani of the middle ear), as well as the mylohyoid and anterior digastric musculature.

Given the role of the trigeminal nerve, it is THE nerve of the dental professional, and any other clinician focusing his or her attention to the head.

It is important to recall that autonomic nerve fibers (both sympathetic and parasympathetic) "hitch a ride" along the various trigeminal nerve branches to reach their target organs and tissues (glands and smooth musculature of the head).

Branches of the Trigeminal Nerve

The specific named branches of V-1, V-2, and V-3 should be reviewed.

The supraorbital, supratrochlear, infratrochlear, and lacrimal nerve from V-1 all originate within the orbit and supply the upper eyelid and forehead. The external nasal nerve also originates from V-1 within the orbit (from nasociliary n.) and serves the bridge of the nose.

The infraorbital branch of V-2 passes out of the infraorbital foramen and supplies the entire midface between the lower eyelid and upper lip. More laterally, the zygomaticofacial and zygomaticotemporal branches of V-2 also serve the midface region.

The buccal and mental branches of V-3 serve the cutaneous tissues overlying the mandible. The auriculotemporal branch of V-3 also serves the upper mandible as well as the cutaneous tissues immediately anterior to the auricle.

The anterosuperior aspect of the nasal cavity is innervated by V-1 fibers. The posteroinferior aspect of the nasal cavity is innervated by V-2 fibers. The nasopharynx is innervated by V-2.

The hard and soft palates are innervated by V-2. The remainder of the oral cavity is innervated by V-3.

The Trigeminal Nerve and the Skull

V-1 passes through the superior orbital fissure, V-2 passes through the foramen rotundum, while V-3 passes through the foramen ovale.

It should be noted that V-3 passes through the foramen ovale within the infratemporal fossa (immediately lateral to the posterior portion of the lateral pterygoid plate).

Study the three-dimensional arrangement of the superior orbital fissure, the foramen rotundum, and the foramen ovale (from superior to inferior).

The superior orbital fissure opens within the orbit. The foramen rotundum opens at the posterior wall of the pterygopalatine fossa. The foramen ovale opens within the roof of the infratemporal fossa.

Maxillary Nerve (V-2)

Recall the location of the pterygomaxillary fissure (between the posterior portion of the maxillary bone and anterior portion of the lateral pterygoid plate). This fissure opens up into the pterygopalatine fossa from a lateral approach.

Recall that V-2 and the pterygopalatine ganglion are found within the pterygopalatine fossa.

V-2 and the nerve of the pterygoid canal (carrying preganglionic parasympathetic fibers and postganglionic sympathetic fibers) enter the pterygopalatine fossa through its posterior wall via the foramen rotundum and the pterygoid canal (respectively). Also in the posterior wall of the pterygopalatine fossa one finds the opening of the pharyngeal canal. Fibers of V-2 leave the fossa via this opening before traveling to the posterior nasopharynx.

Notice specifically the entire course of V-2 as it travels from posterior to anterior through the floor of the orbit and the roof of the maxillary sinus. Its distal-most branch is the infraorbital nerve which you have seen in a previous chapter.

As V-2 passes anteriorly within the roof of the maxillary sinus (as the infraorbital nerve) it gives off three primary branches. These branches are the posterior superior, middle superior, and anterior superior alveolar nerves. These nerves are responsible for innervation of the maxillary portion of the midface and the maxillary teeth.

Notice that the anterior superior alveolar nerve and the middle superior alveolar nerve are quite a distance apart. This occurs as the nerves diverge from each other around the canine fossa. This divergence creates an area with no overlying nervous tissue on the lateral wall of the maxillary sinus. This space may be exploited if the surgeon needs to approach the maxillary sinus via the Caldwell-Luc approach. (1, p. 137)

Given its close proximity with the pterygopalatine ganglion within the pterygopalatine fossa, V-2 provides a means of distribution to both postganglionic parasympathetic and postganglionic sympathetic fibers within the midface region.

At the posterior aspect of the lateral nasal wall one finds the pterygopalatine fossa. The pterygopalatine ganglion can be found within the fossa space. V-2 also passes through this space and the ganglion is attached and connected to V-2. Branches from V-2 (which may pass through the ganglion given its proximity) enter the nasal cavity through the sphenopalatine foramen (within the medial or deep wall of the fossa) to supply the posteroinferior nasal cavity. The branch of V-2 which serves the posteroinferior nasal septum is the nasopalatine nerve. Branches of V-2 also serve the lateral nasal wall and arise from more distal V-2 branches (such as the palatine nerves). The anterior ethmoidal nerve (from the nasociliary nerve in the orbit) serves the anterosuperior nasal septum and lateral nasal wall (via the external nasal nerve branch). Thus V-1 (anterosuperiorly) and V-2 (posteroinferiorly) afferently serve the nasal cavity.

Recall that branches of V-2 from the pterygopalatine fossa travel inferiorly within the palatine canal to reach the posterior portion of the hard palate where they exit (with the palatine arteries) via the greater and lesser palatine foramina. The greater palatine nerve then serves the hard palate anteriorly while the lesser palatine nerve travels posteriorly to serve the soft palate.

Maxillary Artery Review

The maxillary artery lies within the infratemporal fossa space.

Proximal branches of the maxillary artery have already been discussed in previous chapters. Recall that the maxillary artery is serving all the structures of the infratemporal fossa including the muscles of mastication.

As the maxillary artery travels anteriorly it gives off some final branches before its most distal sphenopalatine branch. These branches are the infraorbital, descending palatine, posterior superior alveolar, and buccal branches.

The buccal artery will serve the lateral midface.

The descending palatine artery will travel within the palatine canal (with the greater and lesser palatine nerves) and ultimately serve the hard and soft palates.

The infraorbital artery will travel within the orbital floor.

The posterior superior alveolar artery supplies maxillary molar teeth and the maxillary sinus. The other maxillary teeth are served by middle and anterior superior alveolar arteries which originate from the infraorbital artery within the orbital floor.

Greater and Lesser Petrosal Nerves

The greater and lesser petrosal nerves travel over the floor of the cranial vault.

Note that the greater petrosal nerve is medial to the lesser petrosal nerve. Both nerves are carrying preganglionic parasympathetic fibers. The greater petrosal nerve is carrying these fibers from the facial nerve, while the lesser petrosal nerve is carrying these fibers from the glossopharyngeal nerve. The specifics of these nerves were covered in previous chapters and should be reviewed at this time.

Otic Ganglion:
> The glossopharyngeal nerve (CN IX) arises from the medulla and leaves the skull via the jugular foramen. Its primary role is to afferently serve the posterior portion of the pharynx (the oropharynx, to be specific).

> Immediately following its exit from the skull, a small set of fibers (the tympanic nerve) split off from the glossopharyngeal nerve. These fibers travel superiorly right back up into the skull through the tympanic canaliculus (found directly between the jugular foramen and the carotid canal).

> These preganglionic parasympathetic fibers travel through the middle ear space before leaving the temporal bone of the skull by means of the lesser petrosal nerve through the hiatus for the lesser petrosal nerve. The lesser petrosal nerve then travels over the internal skull base before exiting through the foramen ovale adjacent to the mandibular branch of the trigeminal nerve.

> The preganglionic fibers then synapse in the otic ganglion which is found immediately medial to the trunk of mandibular branch of the trigeminal nerve after it has exited the skull base.

> Postganglionic fibers exit the otic ganglion and hitch a ride on the auriculotemporal nerve before finally jumping off in the substance of the parotid gland to innervate it.

Pterygopalatine Ganglion:
> The facial nerve arises from the pons and leaves the cranial vault via the internal acoustic meatus where it enters temporal bone.

> Within the temporal bone the facial nerve travels both superior and posterior to the middle ear space. Before the facial nerve leaves the temporal bone at the stylomastoid foramen (at which point its fibers are entirely motor efferents) it gives off the greater petrosal nerve and the chorda tympani nerve.

> The greater petrosal nerve carries preganglionic parasympathetic fibers destined for the pterygopalatine fossa. It exits temporal bone (after splitting from the facial nerve) via the hiatus for the greater petrosal nerve.

> The greater petrosal nerve then arrives at the posterior wall of the pterygopalatine ganglion after having exited the skull via the foramen lacerum. These preganglionic parasympathetic fibers join with postganglionic sympathetic fibers (via the deep petrosal nerve) to become the nerve of the pterygoid canal.

The nerve of the pterygoid canal arrives at the pterygopalatine ganglion through the posterior wall of the pterygopalatine fossa. There, the sympathetic fibers pass through (having already synapsed in the superior cervical ganglion), and the parasympathetic fibers synapse with their postganglionic counterparts. Both sets of postganglionic autonomic fibers then "hitch a ride" with the maxillary division of the trigeminal nerve (V-2) as it travels through the inferior orbital floor and maxillary sinus roof. They then jump onto the zygomatic nerve and travel to the lacrimal gland in the orbit. They may arrive at the lacrimal gland directly, or by hitching a ride with V-1 first.

Recall that the postganglionic sympathetic fibers serving the head and neck all originate at the superior cervical ganglion and travel to their target destinations via the internal and external carotid arteries and their branches.

Sources Cited:

1. Brzezinski, et al. Laboratory and Study Guide for Head and Neck Anatomy: Dissection of the Head and Neck. Ann Arbor, MI. 2013

Special Acknowledgment - The image at the end of this chapter was drawn by Dr. Ivan Chicchon and was modeled after the original art by Jaye Schlesinger on p. 138 of Brzezinski, et al. Laboratory and Study Guide for Head and Neck Anatomy: Dissection of the Head and Neck. Ann Arbor, MI. 2013

Laboratory Approach

☐1. Examine the three divisions of the trigeminal nerve with special attention to the maxillary division (V2). Follow the maxillary nerve from its location within the pterygopalatine fossa, through the orbital floor, and out the infraorbital foramen.

☐2. Examine the pterygopalatine fossa. Describe the fossa in relation to the pterygomaxillary fissure and the sphenopalatine foramen as well. Describe which structures traverse the fossa and which structures reside within the fossa.

☐3. Examine the pterygopalatine ganglion. Describe its role in autonomic innervation of the orbit and midface. Describe its preganglionic fibers from the greater petrosal nerve and its postganglionic fibers which travel with regional nerves to reach glandularity of the orbit and midface.

☐4. Examine the third portion of the maxillary artery and its branches.

☐5. Examine the superior dental plexus of nerves and describe their innervation of the maxillary teeth.

☐6. Review the osteology of the orbital floor, maxillary sinus roof, and sphenoid ethmoid, and maxillary bones.

Key Regional Structures

Maxillary a. (third or pterygopalatine portion)
    Posterior superior alveolar a.
    Infraorbital a.
        anterior superior alveolar a.
    Descending palatine a.
        greater palatine a.
        lesser palatine a.
    Artery of pterygoid canal
    Artery of pharyngeal canal
    Sphenopalatine a. (distal-most portion of maxillary a.)

Ophthalmic n. (V1)
Maxillary n. (V2)
    Zygomatic n.
        zygomaticofacial n.
        zygomaticotemporal n.
    Infraorbital n.
        posterior, middle, and anterior superior alveolar nn.
            superior dental plexus of nn.
        gingival branches
        nasal branches
        labial branches
    Palatine nerve trunk
        greater palatine n.
        lesser palatine n.
        posterior inferior lateral nasal n.
    Pharyngeal n. (n. of pharyngeal canal)
    Posterior superior nasal n.
        lateral branches
        medial branches (nasopalatine n.)
Mandibular n. (V3)

Pterygopalatine fossa
Pterygopalatine ganglion

Nerve of the pterygoid canal
    Greater petrosal n. (preganglionic parasympathetic fibers from VII)
    Deep petrosal n. (postganglionic sympathetic fibers from sup. cerv. gang.)

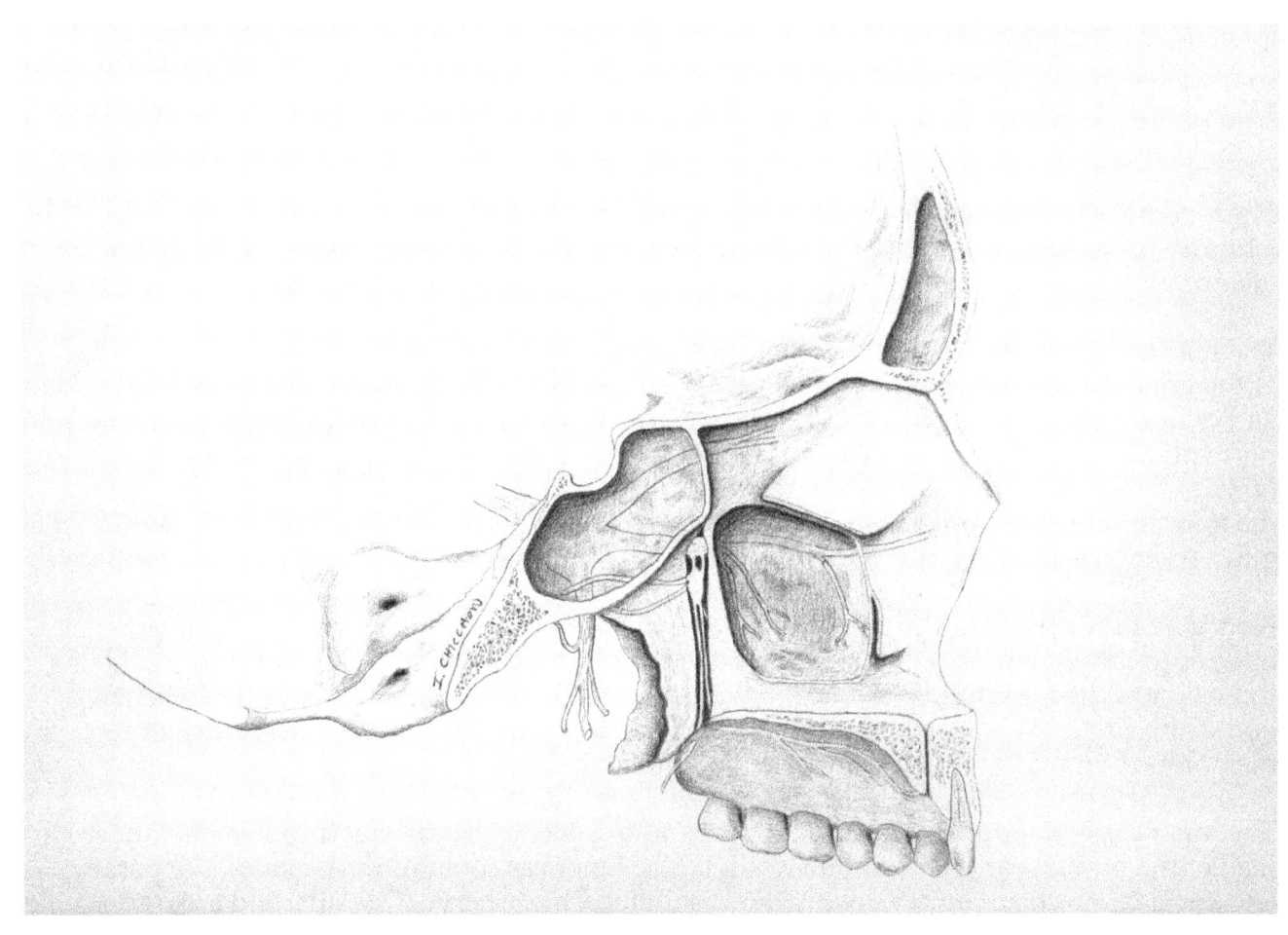

Ear

<u>Introduction</u>

This chapter will primarily cover the middle ear space, but will also review relevant regional structures.

The external ear includes the auricle and external auditory meatus as well as the external auditory tube. The medial (deep) wall of the external ear is the lateral aspect of the tympanic membrane.

The middle ear is a space contained within temporal bone. Its lateral wall is the medial aspect of the tympanic membrane. Its medial (deep) wall is the "window wall" containing the round and oval windows. Anteriorly the middle ear communicates with the nasopharynx via the pharyngotympanic tube. Posteriorly the middle ear communicates with mastoid air spaces (via the mastoid antrum and aditus ad antrum). The promontory of the deep (medial) wall of the middle ear space is the lateral protuberance of the cochlea from the inner ear space into the middle ear space.

Notice that the roof of the middle ear is the tegmen tympani and the space immediately inferior to the roof (within the middle ear) is the epitympanic recess. The middle ear contains three bones (the middle ear "ossicles"), the malleus, the incus, and the stapes. These small bones amplify and control the transmission of sound from vibrations of the tympanic membrane to movement of the liquid endolymph within the inner ear (cochlea).

The inner ear is a space contained within temporal bone. Its lateral wall is the medial (deep) wall of the middle ear (the "window wall"). The inner ear contains the vestibular apparatus and cochlea which are innervated by the vestibulocochlear nerve (CN VIII) and are responsible for balance and hearing (respectively).

Notice that the internal acoustic meatus allows passage of both the facial nerve and the vestibulocochlear nerve into temporal bone. The vestibulocochlear nerve terminates at the inner ear while the facial nerve travels superior and posterior to the middle ear space as its efferent fibers progress toward the stylomastoid foramen.

It should be noted that the mastoid process and the mastoid air cells within the mastoid process reside immediately posterior and inferior to the middle ear space.

The mastoid airspaces communicate with the middle ear space through the posterior wall of the middle ear space.

<u>Middle Ear</u>

The middle ear space lies between the tympanic membrane (the middle ear's lateral wall) and the "window wall" containing the promontory and middle ear windows (the middle ear's medial wall).

Notice that the anterior wall of the middle ear space communicates with the nasopharynx via the auditory tube. The muscles of the soft palate attach to the auditory tube. The levator veli palatini is innervated by the vagus nerve. The tensor veli palatini is innervated efferently by the mandibular division of the trigeminal nerve (V-3).

Originating from the anterior wall of the middle ear (superior to the cartilaginous auditory tube) and sphenoid bone is the tensor tympani muscle. It inserts into the manubrium of the malleus (a middle ear "ossicle") and acts to dampen the vibrations of the tympanic membrane. It is innervated by the mandibular division of the trigeminal nerve (V-3) and is served vascularly by the middle meningeal artery (superior tympanic branch). Recall that the tensor veli palatini is also innervated by V-3. Thus, both the tensors of the head (veli palatini and tympani) are innervated by V-3. This arrangement is as it is due to the fact that both the tensor muscles of the head are derived from the first pharyngeal arch embryologically (thus sharing the same innervation). (1, Muscles of the Head and Neck - Tensor Tympani)

The lateral wall of the middle ear space contains the tympanic membrane. The malleus is attached directly to the tympanic membrane. It articulates with the incus more medially. The incus, in turn, will articulate with the more medially placed stapes.

Notice the chorda tympani nerve (from CN VII) passes from posterior to anterior through the middle ear space between the malleus and the incus. The chorda carries both special afferent fibers (taste from the anterior 2/3 of the tongue) and preganglionic parasympathetic fibers destined for the submandibular ganglion. The sensory (taste) cell bodies of the chorda are located at the geniculate ganglion (at the genu of the facial nerve). Another parasympathetic nerve arises from the facial nerve. It is the greater petrosal nerve, and its preganglionic parasympathetic fibers are destined for the pterygopalatine ganglion.

The medial wall of the middle ear space contains the promontory which represents the protuberance of the inner ear (the cochlea) into the middle ear space. The medial wall is called the "window wall" because it contains the oval and round windows.

The oval window is superoposterior to the promontory on the medial wall of the middle ear and is the site of placement of the footplate of stapes. Sound is transmitted from the tympanic membrane, through the ossicles, and into the inner ear via the footplate of stapes. As stapes moves, its footplate displaces the endolymph of the inner ear through the small oval window. As endolymph moves within the inner ear, a release valve is necessary (since liquid cannot be compressed and the endolymph is enclosed within petrous temporal bone). This release valve is the round window which is located inferoposterior to the promontory on the medial wall of the middle ear.

As the footplate of stapes presses into the inner ear space (via the oval window), the endolymph moves through the cochlea and causes an ever-so-slight "bulging" of the tissues overlying the round window. In this way the oval and round windows allow for the movement of liquid within the cochlea of the inner ear.

The posterior wall of the middle ear contains the pyramid ("pyramidal eminence"). This structure contains muscular fibers attaching to the neck of stapes. These fibers act to dampen the vibrations of stapes and are efferently innervated by the facial nerve (CN VII). These fibers (stapedius fibers) are entirely enclosed within bone and are derived from the second pharyngeal arch embryologically. (2, Muscles of the Head and Neck - Stapedius)

In summary, the middle ear may be though of as a "box":
- The lateral wall of the box is the tympanic membrane.
- The medial wall of the box is the "window wall" containing the oval window, round window, promontory (of the inner ear's cochlea), semicircular canal protuberance, and the protuberance of the facial nerve as it travels superior and posterior to the middle ear space.
- The posterior wall contains the openings to the mastoid air cells, the pyramid (containing stapedius fibers), and the chorda tympani as it arises from the facial nerve posterior to the middle ear.
- The anterior wall contains the tensor tympani muscle and the auditory tube. It also contains nervous fibers leaving the middle ear space (including the chorda tympani fibers and lesser petrosal nerve fibers).

Nerves of the Middle Ear

The facial nerve lies superior and posterior to the middle ear space. The facial nerve only innervates the stapedius muscle in the middle ear region. Its autonomic fibers (via the greater petrosal nerve and chorda tympani) leave the facial nerve as it travels through the temporal bone of the region.

Tympanic nerve fibers overly the promontory of the medial (deep) wall of the middle ear. The tympanic plexus fibers are preganglionic parasympathetic fibers from the glossopharyngeal nerve. These tympanic nerve fibers enter the middle ear space via the tympanic canaliculus. The fibers "separate" and flay out over the promontory before coming back together again as the lesser petrosal nerve fibers. These fibers will ultimately travel to the otic ganglion to serve the parotid gland and have been covered in a previous chapter.

The innervation of the parotid gland (via the glossopharyngeal nerve) should be reviewed at this time. The glossopharyngeal nerve (CN IX) arises from the medulla and leaves the skull via the jugular foramen. Immediately following its exit from the skull, a small set of fibers (the tympanic nerve fibers) split off from the glossopharyngeal nerve. These fibers travel superiorly right back up into the skull through the tympanic canaliculus (found directly between the jugular foramen and the carotid canal). These preganglionic parasympathetic fibers travel through the middle ear space (as the tympanic plexus over the promontory) before leaving the temporal bone of the skull by means of the lesser petrosal nerve. The lesser petrosal nerve then travels over the internal skull base before exiting through the foramen ovale adjacent to the mandibular branch of the trigeminal nerve. The preganglionic fibers then synapse in the otic ganglion which is found immediately medial to the trunk of mandibular branch of the trigeminal nerve after it has exited the skull base. Postganglionic fibers exit the otic ganglion and hitch a ride on the auriculotemporal nerve before finally jumping off in the substance of the parotid gland to innervate it.

<u>Soft Palate Review</u>

The veli palatini muscles are reviewed here due to their regional relationship with the auditory tube.

Recall that the tensor veli palatini arises from the anterolateral aspect of the tube whereas the levator veli palatini arises from the posteromedial aspect of the tube.

The tensor veli palatini originates from the scaphoid fossa (sphenoid bone) and the lateral wall of the auditory tube cartilage. It inserts into the palatine aponeurosis after passing around the hamular hook of the medial pterygoid plate. It acts to tense the soft palate (thus its name) and open the auditory tube. It is served by V3 and the ascending pharyngeal artery. The tensor veli palatini muscle's primary job is to keep the soft palate taut and to open the auditory tube. (3, Muscles of the Head and Neck - Tensor Veli Palatini)

The levator veli palatini originates from the apex of the petrous portion of the temporal bone and the medial wall of the auditory tube cartilage. It inserts into the musculature and fascia of the soft palate as well as the palatine aponeurosis. It acts to elevate the soft palate (thus its name) and is served by the vagus nerve and the ascending pharyngeal artery. (4, Muscles of the Head and Neck - Levator Veli Palatini)

The superior-most muscle of the soft palate is the palatopharyngeus. It originates from the bony palate and inserts into the posterior wall of the pharynx and the posterior margin of the thyroid cartilage. It acts to elevate the larynx and is served by the vagus nerve and the ascending pharyngeal artery. (5, Muscles of the Head and Neck - Palatopharyngeus)

Sources Cited:

1-5. Gest, et al. Anatomy Tables (electronic MedCharts). Ann Arbor, MI. 2000

Laboratory Approach

☐1. Examine the auricle (external ear) and the external auditory canal. Describe their relationship to the TMJ.

☐2. Examine the walls of the middle ear and specific structures on each wall. Describe which deeper structures contribute to the formation of certain middle ear wall structures (when relevant).

☐3. Examine the auditory ossicles and describe their function in hearing.

☐4. Examine the two muscles of the middle ear, their innervation, and function.

☐5. Examine the course of the facial nerve through the temporal bone over and behind the middle ear. Describe its two autonomic branches.

☐6. Examine all of the nerves which enter and exit the middle ear space (CN VII, VIII, and IX). Describe where they come from, go to, and the functions they serve.

Key Regional Structures

Middle Ear

    Bony chambers
        Tympanic cavity
        Epitympanic recess
        Mastoid antrum
           aditus ad antrum
        Mastoid air cells

    Foramina and openings
        Internal acoustic meatus
        External acoustic meatus
        Petrotympanic fissure
        Inferior Tympanic canaliculus
        Hiatus (& groove) for greater petrosal n.
        Hiatus (& groove) for lesser petrosal n.
        Stylomastoid foramen
        Carotid canal
        Jugular fossa & foramen
        Oval (vestibular) window
        Round (cochlear) window

    Bony contours and structures
        Petrous ridge
        Tegmen tympani
        Arcuate eminence
        Anterior (superior) semicircular canal
        Promontory
        Cochlea
        Bony auditory canal
        Semicanal for the tensor tympani m.

    Auditory ossicles
        Malleus
           anterior process & head
           tensor tympani m.
        Incus
           body; short and long processes
        Stapes
           head
           stapedius m. & tendon
        Tympanic membrane

Nerves
      Vestibulocochlear n. (CN VIII)
      Facial n. (CN VII)
        geniculate ganglion
        greater petrosal n.
        chorda tympani
      Glossopharyngeal n. (CN IX)
        tympanic br.
        lesser petrosal n.
        tympanic plexus

Fascial Spaces

Introduction

Many important structures in the head and neck are invested within a fascial sheet. These fascial sheets create various compartments. These fascial sheets also create planes between invested structures and compartments. While anatomically important, these sheets, compartments, and planes are also clinically important. Just as fascial compartments serve to localize normal anatomic structures, fluids such as exudates or extravasated blood may similarly be localized to various fascial compartments in circumstances of pathology. These fluids (or other pathologic materials or organisms) may subsequently spread to adjacent fascial spaces and compartments by breaking through fascial boundaries. Knowledge of how this spreading occurs is important in the treatment of abscesses or other pathology.

Earlier in this text certain fascial spaces were examined in detail. These included the parotid fossa, the submandibular and paralingual spaces, the prevertebral and retropharyngeal spaces, and the carotid sheath. The midface and mandible are also invested with a complex series of fascial sheets. The most important of these are the masticator space and the lateral pharyngeal space. This chapter will carefully examine these two spaces. This chapter will also review the carotid sheath (a.k.a. the retrostyloid space).

It should be noted that this chapter is modeled after the "Fascial Spaces" chapter in Brzezinski, et al. Laboratory and Study Guide for Head and Neck Anatomy: Dissection of the Head and Neck. Ann Arbor, MI. 2013. The Masticator Space, Lateral Pharyngeal Space, and Carotid Sheath sections are reworded from this source with the permission of the most recent contributors (Brzezinski and Cortright).

Masticator Space

The masticator space is a collection of compartments comprised of fascia surrounding the ramus of the mandible and the muscles of mastication. This space can be further broken up. The individual spaces which collectively combine to create the masticator space are as follows:

I. Superficial Masticator Compartment:
   A. Temporal Space
        This space is typically subdivided into superficial and deep spaces. The superficial temporal space lies deep to the temporal fascia and superficial to the muscular fascia of the temporalis muscle. This superficial space typically contains a process of the buccal fat pad and thus communicates with the buccal space. The deep temporal space lies between the periosteum of the lateral surface of the bony temporal fossa and the muscular fascia investing the temporalis muscle. It is essentially the temporalis muscular compartment.

B. Masseteric Space

This space is contained by the fascia of the masseter muscle. Its deep surface is adjacent to the lateral surface of the mandibular ramus and extends superiorly to the temporal fascia above the zygomatic arch. It is essentially the masseteric muscular compartment.

II. Arthro-osseus Compartment

This space is contained by the periosteum of the mandibular ramus and the joint capsule of the temporomandibular joint. Its posterior boundary is the posterior border of the mandibular ramus, and its anterior border is the edge of the anterior-most attachment of the pterygomasseteric sling. This space is separate from that around the body of the mandible inferoanteriorly with distinct boundaries.

III. Intermediate Compartment

A. Lateral Pterygoid Space

This space is contained by the muscular fascia of the lateral pterygoid muscle (superior and inferior heads) and its bony attachments. It is essentially the lateral pterygoid muscular compartment.

B. Pterygomandibular Space

This space is found medial to the ramus of the mandible, inferior to the lateral pterygoid muscular fascia and superior to the medial pterygoid muscular fascia.

Importantly, branches of V3 and the maxillary artery pass through this space. As such, this is the space where anesthetic intended to block the inferior alveolar and lingual nerves is deposited.

IV. Deep Masticator Compartment (a.k.a. Medial Pterygoid Space)

This space is contained by the muscular fascia of the medial pterygoid muscle and its bony attachments. It is essentially the medial pterygoid muscular compartment. Note that the interpterygoid fascia consists of the fascia covering the lateral side of the medial pterygoid muscle, while the fascia covering the medial side of the medial pterygoid muscle forms part of the lateral wall of the lateral pharyngeal space.

Lateral Pharyngeal Space

The lateral pharyngeal space lies posterolateral to the fascia of the pharynx, posteromedial to the fascia of the masticator apparatus (ramus of the mandible and pterygoid musculature), and anterior to the carotid sheath. Superiorly, the space is bounded by the base of the skull. Anteriorly, the space is bounded by the fusion of the fascia of the lateral pharyngeal wall and the muscular fascia of the medial pterygoid muscle. Posteriorly, the space is bounded by the stylomandibular membrane and the muscular fascia of the styloid musculature which fuses with the fascia of the lateral pharyngeal wall. Inferiorly, a sheet of fascia between the styloglossus muscle and base of the mandibular ramus bound the space. Medially it is bounded by the hyoid bone and its attachments.

Clinically, the inferior boundary of this space is the location typically chosen for surgical drainage (immediately inferomedial to the attachment of the medial pterygoid muscle).

Dr. John Lillie, whose work in "A Dental Student's Guide to Dissection of the Human Body" was the model for "Laboratory and Study Guide for Head and Neck Anatomy: Dissection of the Head and Neck", wrote that the lateral pharyngeal space is a key space of the head and neck because it communicates with six other fascial spaces (parotid, masticator, retropharyngeal, retrostyloid, submandibular, and paralingual) and is the main highway through which perioral infections may gain access to the deep neck and mediastinum.

Carotid Sheath (a.k.a. Retrostyloid Space)

This space is bounded anteriorly by the fascial investment of the sternocleidomastoid muscle (inferiorly) and the styloid process and styloid musculature (superiorly). It is bounded posteriorly by the prevertebral fascia. It is lateroposterior to the lateral pharyngeal space and medioposterior to the deepest portion of the parotid fossa.

The fascial investment of the carotid sheath itself is essentially a tube of loose connective tissue surrounding the common carotid artery, the internal jugular vein, and the vagus nerve.

Sources Cited:

Brzezinski, et al. Laboratory and Study Guide for Head and Neck Anatomy: Dissection of the Head and Neck. Ann Arbor, MI. 2013

☐1. Review and examine the parotid fossa, the submandibular and paralingual spaces, the prevertebral and retropharyngeal spaces.

☐2. Examine the masticator space and its subdivisions. Describe the anatomic boundaries of each.

☐3. Examine the lateral pharyngeal space. Describe its anatomic boundaries and relationships to all adjacent spaces.

☐4. Review the carotid sheath, its boundaries, and its relationship to adjacent spaces.

☐5. Describe the spread of infection from each space to adjacent spaces as well as to the mediastinum.

Parotid gland fossa
Submandibular space
Paralingual space
Prevertebral space
Retropharyngeal space
Masticator space
      Superficial compartment
        temporal (superficial & deep) space
        masseteric space
      Arthro-osseous compartment
      Intermediate compartment
        lateral pterygoid space
        pterygomandibular space
      Deep compartment (medial pterygoid space)
Lateral pharyngeal space
Retrostyloid space (superior extent of the carotid sheath)

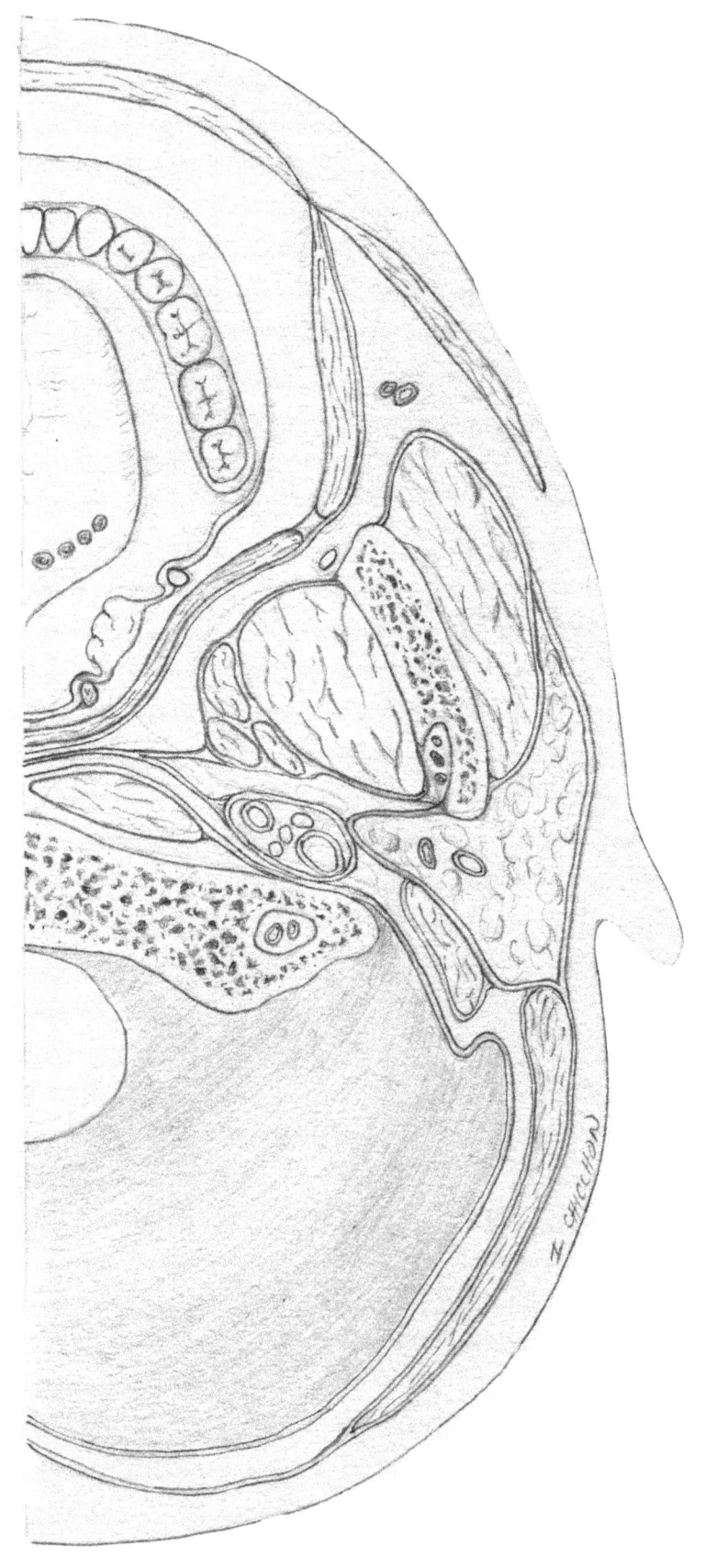

Appendix: Summary of Bony Openings

LOCATION	OPENING	CONTENTS
ANTERIOR CRANIAL FOSSA (Cribriform plate of ethmoid bone)	OLFACTORY FORAMINA	Olfactory nn. (CN I)
ANTERIOR CRANIAL FOSSA (In lesser wing of sphenoid bone)	OPTIC CANAL	Optic n. (CN II) Ophthalmic a.
MIDDLE CRANIAL FOSSA (Between lesser & greater wings of sphenoid bone)	SUPERIOR ORBITAL FISSURE	Oculomotor n. (CN III) Trochlear n. (CN IV) 3 branches of ophthalmic n. (CN V$_1$): Frontal n. Lacrimal n. Nasociliary n. Abducens n. (CN VI) Superior ophthalmic v.
MIDDLE CRANIAL FOSSA	*FORAMEN ROTUNDUM	Maxillary n. (CN V$_2$)
MIDDLE CRANIAL FOSSA	FORAMEN OVALE	Mandibular n. (CN V$_3$) Lesser petrosal n. (Br. of CN IX) Accessory meningeal a. (inconstant)
MIDDLE CRANIAL FOSSA	FORAMEN SPINOSUM	Middle meningeal a.
MIDDLE CRANIAL FOSSA (Post. to foramen lacerum)	CAROTID CANAL (upper opening) (see also SKULL BASE- CAROTID CANAL, below)	Internal carotid artery Sympathetic fibers (Internal carotid n.)
MIDDLE CRANIAL FOSSA (Immediately lateral to body of sphenoid)	FORAMEN LACERUM (Plugged by cartilage in life)	Emissary v. connecting pterygoid venous plexus & cavernous sinus
MIDDLE CRANIAL FOSSA (Sup. surface of petrous temporal bone)	HIATUS FOR GR. PETROSAL N. HIATUS FOR LESS. PETROSAL N.	Greater petrosal n. (Br. of CN VII) Lesser petrosal n. (Br. of CN IX)
POSTERIOR CRANIAL FOSSA (Below petrous ridge)	INTERNAL ACOUSTIC MEATUS	Facial n. (CN VII) Vestibulocochlear n. (CN VIII)
POSTERIOR CRANIAL FOSSA (Inferior to internal acoustic meatus, at end of sulcus for sigmoid sinus)	JUGULAR FORAMEN (see also SKULL BASE- JUGULAR FOSSA, below)	Transition from inferior petrosal & sigmoid sinus to internal jugular v Glossopharyngeal n. (CN IX) Vagus n. (CN X) Accessory n. (CN XI)
POSTERIOR CRANIAL FOSSA (In lateral wall of foramen magnum, above occipital condyle)	HYPOGLOSSAL CANAL	Hypoglossal n. (CN XII)
CALVARIA (Lateral to sagittal suture near lambdoidal suture)	PARIETAL FORAMEN	Parietal emissary v.

Appendix: Summary of Bony Openings

LOCATION	OPENING	CONTENTS
SKULL BASE (At posterior end of occipital condyle)	CONDYLOID CANAL	Condylar emissary v. (inconstant)
SKULL BASE (Posterior to styloid process; lateral to jugular fossa)	STYLOMASTOID FORAMEN	Facial n. (CN VII) Stylomastoid a.
SKULL BASE (Posterior to mastoid process)	MASTOID FORAMEN	Mastoid emissary v.
SKULL BASE	FORAMEN MAGNUM	Spinal cord/medulla Meninges Vertebral aa. Ant. & post. spinal aa. Spinal roots of accessory n. (CN XI)
SKULL BASE (Medial to styloid process)	JUGULAR FOSSA	Superior bulb of internal jugular v.
SKULL BASE (Anteromedial to jugular fossa)	CAROTID CANAL (lower opening)	Internal carotid a. Sympathetic fibers (Internal carotid n.)
SKULL BASE (On bony ridge between jugular fossa & carotid canal)	INFERIOR TYMP. CANALICULUS	Tympanic n. (Br. of CN IX)
SKULL BASE (In sphenoid bone, at anterior edge of foramen lacerum)	*PTERYGOID CANAL	A., v. & n. of pterygoid canal greater petrosal n. (Br. of CN VII) deep petrosal n. (sympathetic)
SKULL BASE (Just above choana, where medial pterygoid plate meets base of vomer)	*PHARYNGEAL CANAL	Pharyngeal a., v. & n. (Br. of CN V_2)
SKULL BASE (Posterior to mandibular fossa)	PETROTYMPANIC FISSURE	Chorda tympani (Br. of CN VII)
HARD PALATE (Anterior midline)	INCISIVE FOSSA (CANAL)	Nasopalatine n. (Br. of CN V_2) Septal br.-sphenopalatine a., v.
HARD PALATE (Medial to M^3)	GREATER PALATINE FORAMEN	Greater palatine a., v. & n. (Br. of CN V_2)
HARD PALATE (Posterior to greater palatine f.)	LESSER PALATINE FORAMEN	Lesser palatine a., v. & n. (Br. of CN V_2)
NASAL CAVITY (Posterior to attached edge of middle concha)	SPHENOPALATINE FORAMEN	Sphenopalatine a. & v. Post. sup. lat. nasal n. (Br. of CN V_2) Nasopalatine n. (Br. of CN V_2)

Appendix: Summary of Bony Openings

LOCATION	OPENING	CONTENTS
MANDIBLE (On medial surface of ramus)	MANDIBULAR FORAMEN	Inferior alveolar a.,v.,n. (Br. of CN V_3)
MANDIBLE	MENTAL FORAMEN	Mental a.,v.,n. (Br. of CN V_3)
ORBIT (On medial wall)	ANT. & POST. ETHMOIDAL FORAMINA	Ant. & post. ethmoidal a.,v.,n. (Br. of CN V_1)
ORBIT (Posterior orbit)	INFERIOR ORBITAL FISSURE	Anastomoses between pterygoid plexus & inferior ophthalmic v.
ORBIT (Lateral wall)	ZYGOMATICOORBITAL FORAMEN	Zygomatic n. (Br. of CN V_2)
FACIAL SKELETON (Anterior surface of zygomatic bone)	ZYGOMATICOFACIAL FORAMEN	Zygomaticofacial n. (Br. of zygomatic n.)
FACIAL SKELETON (Posterior surface of zygomatic bone)	ZYGOMATICOTEMPORAL FOR.	Zygomaticotemporal n. (Br.-zygomatic n.)
FACIAL SKELETON (Superior margin of orbit)	SUPRAORBITAL FOR. (NOTCH)	Supraorbital a., v. & n. (Br. of CN V_1)
FACIAL SKELETON (Inferior margin of orbit)	INFRAORBITAL FORAMEN (GROOVE, CANAL)	Infraorbital a., v. & n. (Br. of CN V_2)
FACIAL SKELETON (Maxillary tuberosity)	POST. SUP. ALVEOLAR FORAMINA	Post. sup. alveolar aa., vv., nn. (Br. of CN V_2)

*SPHENOID SPECIALIZATIONS
   FORAMEN ROTUNDUM
   PTERYGOID CANAL
   PHARYNGEAL CANAL

    These three canals/openings all open anteriorly into a very important space called the PTERYGOPALATINE FOSSA. This fossa can be easily seen from a lateral view of the skull through the PTERYGOMAXILLARY FISSURE which is the narrow entrance (a two-dimensional doorway) between the maxillary tuberosity (the rounded posterior surface of the maxilla) and the anterior edge of the lateral pterygoid plate. The pterygopalatine fossa is important because the maxillary nerve (V_2) enters it via the foramen rotundum, and the major branches of the maxillary nerve originate in the fossa before traveling to their various destinations including most of the deep mid-face (oral and nasal regions) and the maxillary teeth. The pterygoid canal allows autonomic nerve fibers to reach the pterygopalatine ganglion within the pterygopalatine fossa. The pharyngeal canal (the most inferiorly located of these canals) is very small and conveys its neurovascular bundle posteriorly from the fossa into the mucosa lining the uppermost part of the nasopharynx.

NOTE: Much of the information in this appendix was compiled by Dr. Jerry Cortright who generously gave his permission for its use and publication within this text.

ABOUT THE AUTHOR

David W. Brzezinski is a physician who teaches human gross anatomy at the University of Michigan Medical School and School of Dentistry. He directs multiple medical student, dental student, and resident head and neck courses. His interests are primarily basic science relating to the head and neck. He has multiple adjunct appointments with other institutions and has consulted on the curriculum development of dental schools across the United States.

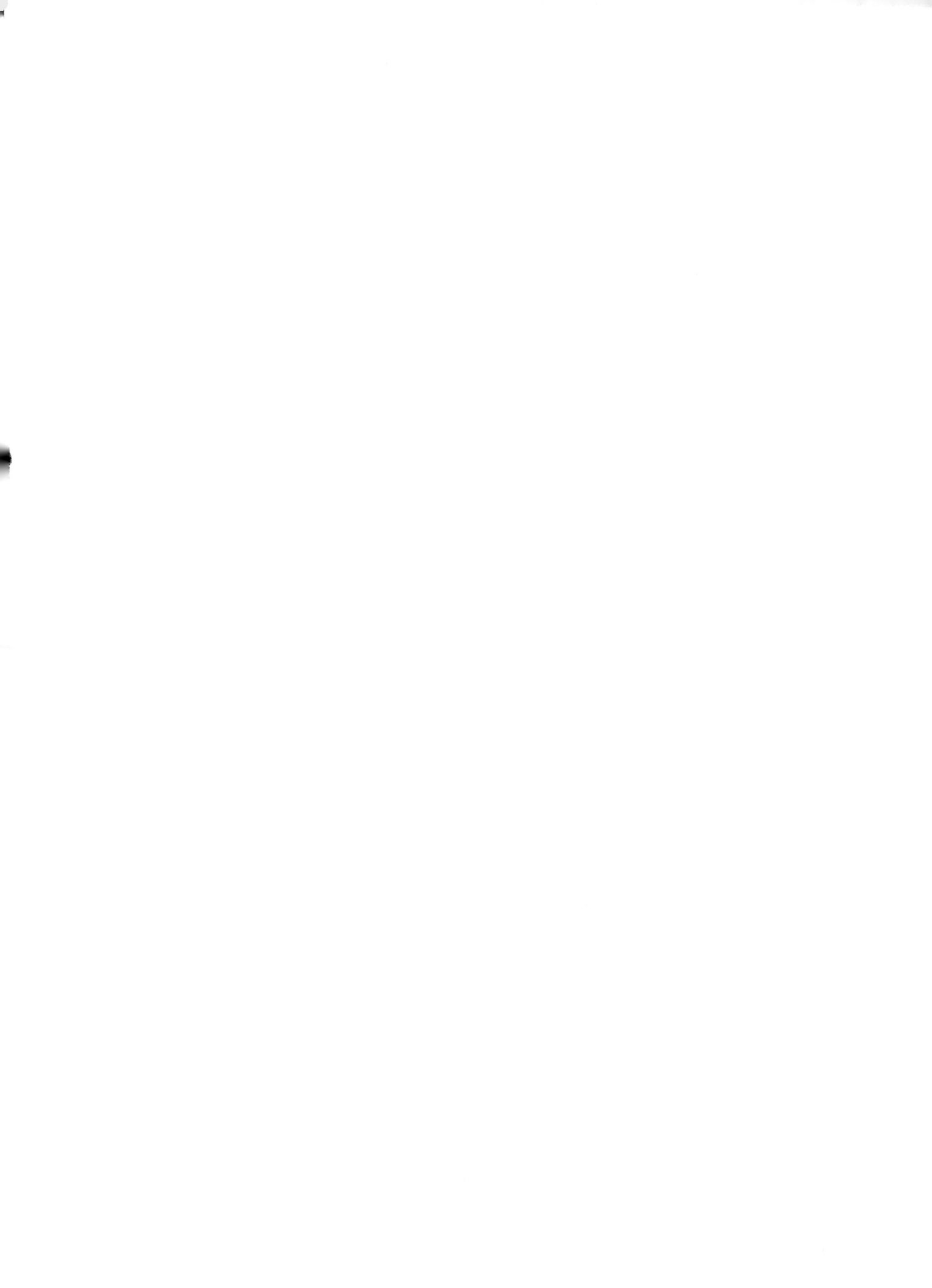